Generis
PUBLISHING

Trauma and religious faith

Kate Miriam Loewenthal

Copyright © 2022 Kate Miriam Loewenthal
Copyright © 2022 Generis Publishing

All rights reserved. This book or any portion thereof may not be reproduced or used in any manner whatsoever without the written permission of the publisher except for the use of brief quotations in a book review.

Title: Trauma and religious faith

ISBN: 979-8-88676-417-8

Author:Kate Miriam Loewenthal

Cover image: www.pixabay.com

Publisher: Generis Publishing
Online orders: www.generis-publishing.com
Contact email: info@generis-publishing.com

Contents

Autobiographical Introduction and Special Thanks 7

EMDR ARTICLES AND CONFERENCE PAPERS. 20

Paper 1: Loewenthal, K.M. (2019) EMDR - Eye Movement Desensitization and Reprocessing therapy and religious faith among orthodox Jewish (*hareidi*) women. *Israel Journal of Psychiatry & Related Sciences, 56 (2), 20-27.* מס \טיפול בתנועות עיניים ואתונה דתית בקרב נשים יהודיות חרדיות. 21

Paper 2: Loewenthal, K.M. (2019) Trauma and therapy: The loss and recovery of faith: An enquiry into experiences. Presented to the *World Psychiatric Association*, Jerusalem, December 2, 2019. 44

Paper 3. Loewenthal, K.M. (2021) Religion, spirituality and recovery from trauma via EMDR therapy. Paper given at the conference of the *International Association for the Psychology of Religion* (online), August 2021..54

Paper 4. Loewenthal, K. (2022) Religious change and posttraumatic growth following trauma therapy: A systematic review. *Mental Health, Religion & Culture,* 63

Paper 5. Loewenthal, K.M. (2022) Religious experiences reported during trauma therapy A paper given at the Psychopathology and Religious Experience Symposium, Saltaire/Leeds University, April 2022..72

FINAL SECTION OF MONOGRAPH: CONCLUSIONS AND QUESTIONS.....................89

REFERENCES...91

APPENDIX 99

Autobiographical Introduction and Special Thanks

Viktor Frankel wrote "I have no statistics, but my own impression…that in Auschwitz more people recovered their belief…" (see Frankl, 2020, p141).

This monograph addresses this issue. Is the overall effect of bad happenings an increase in spirituality?

On a beautiful sunny afternoon, walking across Clapton Common in North London, an area with a large Hasidic Jewish population, I was stopped by a young Hasidic woman "Remember me?" She asked. "Of course", I replied. She had been one of the first volunteers from the Hasidic community to agree to try out a novel (for the community) form of trauma therapy, EMDR. "How are you?" I asked. "I must tell you", she said, "that since I had had that therapy, my *bitachon* has become much stronger". She mentioned how much better she felt, in general, since the therapy, and then returned to the topic of her improved *bitachon*. We had a bit of a discussion on the distinctions between *emunah* (intellectual belief) and *bitachon* (emotional trust). She told me how valuable it was to her that her faith, which had been shaken by the traumatic experiences she had undergone, had become much stronger and more reassuring since her successful trauma therapy.

I was delighted and very intrigued. I began to ask my other therapy clients if they had had a similar experience. More details will follow later in this monograph, but yes – in brief- most other clients experienced a strengthening of religious faith following their recovery from trauma.

Was this the result of EMDR? Perhaps yes, but if so, how? And how might my clients' experiences relate to those of other people experiencing so-called post-traumatic growth? And, a much bigger question, what can we make of Viktor Frankl's suggestion, that people *still* undergoing the most horrific unimaginable traumata, experience a recovery of faith?

What on earth am I doing, an 80-year-old great-grandmother, asking these questions and looking for scientific answers, when much of my time is occupied with a rather contrasting activity: saying psalms *(tehilim)* for the welfare of many people, both in my family and otherwise? And I do a bit of cooking as well, and I love to spend time with my family.

My husband and I have 11 wonderful children, and I am still puzzled as to how I combined motherhood with a Hasidic lifestyle, and full-time employment as an academic psychologist. My academic career included the development of a successful research programme on the scientific study of religious activity and religious feeling and their effects. I had significant encouragement and blessing from the well-known religious leader, the Lubavitcher Rebbe, Rabbi Menachem Mendel Schneerson, and enormous support from many other people. Chief among these is my husband, Dr Naftali Loewenthal, a prominent teacher and scholar of Hasidic philosophy.

I finished my PhD in 1967, in University College London, patiently supervised by the brilliant and very amiable Peter Wason. My thesis looked at the effects of speaking on the way we think…I was concerned with the likelihood that we do not just simply think of what we are going to say, and then say it. What we say has an effect on what we think. I was appointed to a junior academic post (assistant lectureship) in the University of Wales, in Bangor, North Wales. The head of the Psychology department was then Tim Miles, and original and inspiring leader. We rented a cottage on the edge of Snowdonia, a favourite part of the UK, with a view into the Nant Ffrancon valley.

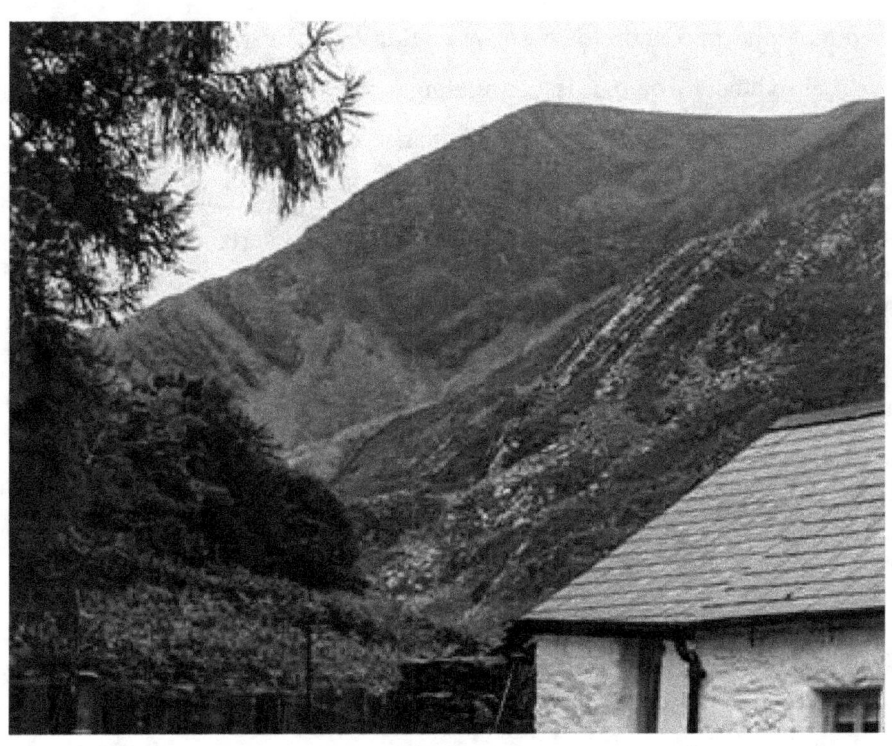

A cottage on the edge of Snowdonia.

We lived there for two years, and did not really want to leave. However our lovely daughter Esther had been born. We experienced all the excitement and amazement of birth directly for the first time, and then came actual parenthood! Quite an adjustment in this case, as Esther was blessed with the ability to get by with very very little sleep. I realised this would be a wonderful gift for her in adulthood, but I certainly found it hard to cut my sleep allowance back to 4 or 5 hours out of 24. The responsibilities also brought home to us the knowledge that the requisites of an observant Jewish life were going to increase. It was already somewhat complicated in the Welsh mountains, with an exciting weekly wait for our kosher meat to arrive from Manchester. It usually got to us in time, but not quite always…freezers were not a norm in those days so we couldn't keep a stock of kosher meat. We realised there would be issues relating to observant Jewish life other than simply the kosher meat supply, particularly of course Jewish education for our children. So with some regrets we packed up and returned to London, saving the beauties of Wales for our vacations. It was certainly hard to leave!

My husband Tali resumed his academic studies. He had registered in University College London to do a psychology degree, and that is where we met. But he abandoned psychology and resumed his study of Judaism when we returned to London from Wales, registering first for a degree in Jewish Studies in University College London, then a PhD, and has remained in the Jewish Studies department at UCL with a Fellowship, alongside a great deal of energetic work on behalf of Chabad. In academia, he specialises in the history of Hasidism and Hasidic mysticism, and also offers a course on Maimonides, and lectures on Jewish philosophy.

I had a lectureship in Psychology in the City University (which later joined the University of London). At City I resumed friendships from undergraduate days at UCL, particularly with Steve Miller and his wife, Liz (a medical researcher), and others. The Millers have remained friends ever since, though I am not very good at keeping up a regular contact.

City had been a Polytechnic, and in the 1960s had a status in the university hierarchy similar to the "new" and "red-brick" universities of that time. They still had to prove that they were as good as the longer-established universities, or indeed (if possible) better. Their members – staff and students – were often self-conscious about whether they belonged to a "good" university. The university's main building is a striking late-Victorian creation in the City (of London). I was very happy there, but…

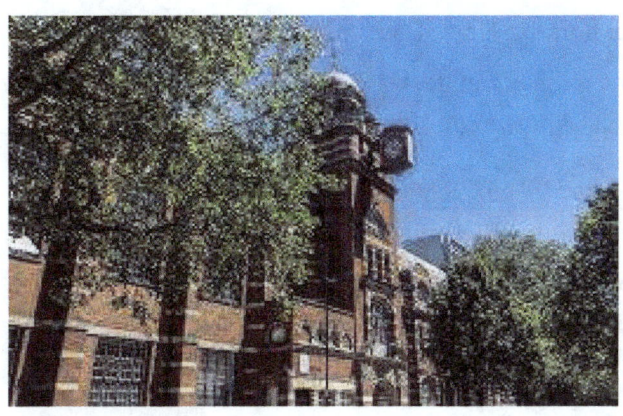

City, University of London.

I'm a bit ashamed to admit that I had my eyes wide open for a post in London university, and was very happy and grateful to find one in Bedford College, London University. This college no longer exists, and its beautiful site and buildings in Regent's Park are now occupied by Regent's College/university. But when I moved there in 1972 there were no omens of the changes to come when London University was restructured in the mid 1980s.

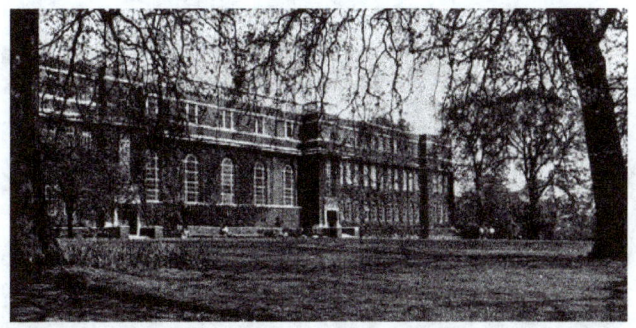

Bedford College, London University, in the 1960s.

When that restructuring happened, Bedford College merged with Royal Holloway College – quite a journey. From 1972-1985, I happily commuted to Regents Park from our home in North London's Stamford Hill. From 1985 until I retired in 2007, my main commute was to Royal Holloway's beautiful but rather distant site in Surrey. When the psychology department first moved there was a collective effort to exaggerate the difficulties of getting there with colleagues telling mock-grim tales of getting lost in the wilds of Surrey, failing to arrive on time. I had to admit that the commute was worth it, a really beautiful campus. And the original building is now appreciated as an exceptional piece of Victorian architecture, although in the 1980s many people thought it was weird, florid, overdone. That opinion is hard to appreciate nowadays, I think, and the college probably owes major gratitude to John Betjeman, the poet Laureate and a leading scion of the arts, who all along was a very outspoken enthusiast for the architecture of Royal Holloway. Betjeman certainly helped to turn what was honestly a tide of scorn into generally universal admiration.

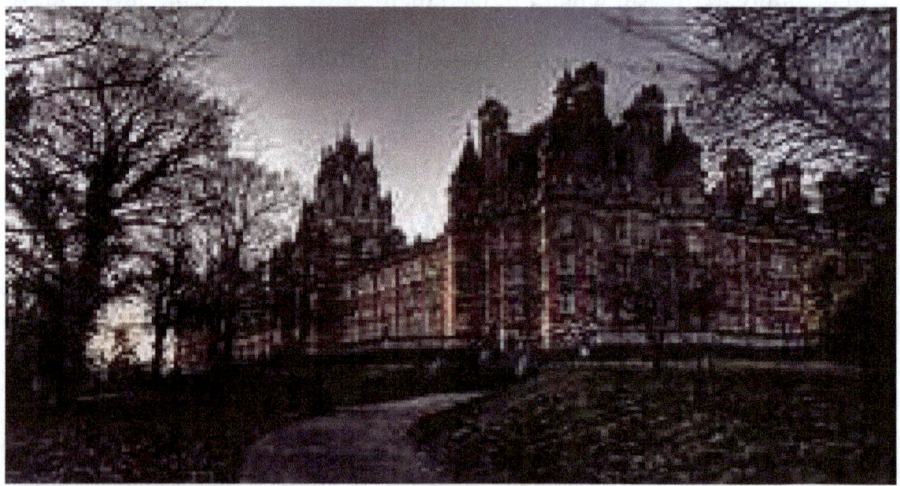

Royal Holloway, University of London – its full name is now Royal Holloway and Bedford New College, University of London.

The pictures above all contain trees, with a reason. I know I find it difficult to get through a day without its dose of green, preferably a walk involving trees. Perhaps this is a result of my upbringing in the countryside on the edge of Guildford, though some people might say we all need green in our lives. Well, I certainly do, every day please! And I certainly appreciate trees in and around my home, and my places of work.

I worked full-time in the universities mentioned above, and came across some misogyny. This was not universal, but it happened. The most memorable example was in an interview for a job I did not get. I was obviously pregnant at the time, and the head of the psychology department looked very sourly – so it seemed to me – and said very sourly – or so it seemed to me: "Do you intend to pursue a (ahem) (an obviously sneering "polite" cough) normal academic career? I said that was my hope, but clearly I hadn't communicated my optimism well enough. I wasn't offered an appointment at that university. It survived, and so (tG) did I. A more light-hearted example came from a colleague who was concerned about the consequences of repeated pregnancies – "You know Kate", he said when I was expecting our tenth child" "Ten tens are a hundred". Another related example was from one of my bosses – who I suppose should remain nameless, though he was a wonderful boss and I believe meant well when contemplating my seventh pregnancy. "Kate" he said, "If you keep on like this you'll ruin your career". I said I hoped my career would not be ruined, and in retrospect wondered whether his comment was some kind of threat. I knew, and knew he knew, that I was a "good egg" – that was quoted to me by a colleague as the boss's opinion. I took great care not to miss teaching a single class on account of pregnancy and childbirth and childcare, I published articles and books, gained research money and attracted good doctoral students at rates rather well above average, and I did not want to be seen as expecting my colleagues to be taking on extra work as a result of my taking a lot of maternity leave. At one point I consulted the great Jewish religious leader, the Lubavitcher Rebbe, and said I was worried about a conflict between my family commitments and my academic commitments. I was quite prepared to abandon academia at that point – it was shortly before our fourth child was due to be born, and I was feeling pressured. I had given up the idea of pursuing a "career" (whatever that meant), and simply felt I should try to do my job as well as possible. The Rebbe's response to my question was: "There is no conflict between Psychology and Torah". I wasn't sure what that implied in terms of my work situation. There were several prominent rabbis associated with the Rebbe, who assisted with his massive workload, so I rushed into their office and asked Rabbi Klein what the Rebbe's reply meant for me: could I/should I resign my academic post? I can't now quote his exact words, but the reply was clear, encouraging, and to the effect that I could and should continue in academia. So I did continue, and I doubt that I would have had the temerity to continue without that encouragement and blessing from the Lubavitcher Rebbe.

I should add that aside from the relatively tiny doses of misogyny, I experienced a lot of kindness and generous support from colleagues, and remember all with gratitude and warmth.

So, after the decision to continue in academia, what next? Shortly after this decision, I encountered my boss passing along the university corridor in Bedford College. "Ah Kate" he said, "You're religious, aren't you?" "Sure," I responded. "Well I have just met this very nice man, Hywel Lewis, who is Professor of Philosophy of Religion in Kings College. I'm sure you'll get on well with him. He's looking for someone to teach the Psychology of

Religion at Kings, where he runs the degree in Religious Studies." "One problem," said I, "I don't know a thing about the Psychology of Religion" "No problem" said the boss. With a flourish he took out a book which he had tucked under his arm. "It's all in here, you'll soon pick it up". The book was by – or at least edited by - Laurie Brown, who had completed his PhD in Bedford College (my employer) some years previously. The book was published by Penguin, which to my mind indicated that it met certain criteria of both interest and intellectual respectability. With this book transferred to my ownership, instructions to phone Hywel Lewis, and a silent resolution to read a little more than simply the contents of Laurie Brown's book, I set off to complete a pleasant and successful interview at King's College. Yes, academic appointments were made rather painlessly and casually at that time, in the early 1970s – at least this was true for part-time appointments (which this was). I needed to construct a brand new (for me) course in the Psychology of Religion for the students of Kings College. Every Thursday afternoon (in term time) for the next twenty years, I taught this course, alongside my full-time activities at Bedford and Royal Holloway, and venturing into the Psychology of Religion revolutionised my academic activities. I was quite busy enough with my teaching and research at Bedford College, and with my growing family, but the incorporation of the religion course into my activities forced me to some conclusions, and changed the focus of my research.

Looking at my list of published academic articles (which I have put in this book's appendix), as well as conference talks (which I haven't included in the appendix), it's pretty clear that I was focused on the social psychology of speech and language until the early 1970s. Thereafter, is a pretty abrupt change to research involving religion.

Religion, I realised, is a pretty important feature of human life – even though in Western countries the proportion of the non-religious are reported to be rising, the majority of people worldwide are religiously identified: 84% according to the Washington Times summary of a major survey by the Pew Centre (Harper, December 2012). Nearly two-thirds identify with non-Christian religions. You wouldn't have the faintest idea that religion was even remotely important or significant to human thinking, feeling or behaviour if you opened any kind of psychology book or journal, unless it was one of the very tiny minority focussing on religion. Very often the term "religion" wasn't and still isn't included in the topic index included at the end of most psychology texts. Typically, hundreds of topics are listed, but religion…no way. If you did find a religion-focused psychology book or journal, you would find that most research was on Westerners, usually North Americans, who were Christian, usually Protestant, and middle-class, usually university students or graduates. Sometimes the research participants were classified as Judeo-Christian. I felt this grouping – Judeo-Christian - was rather mysterious and poorly-defined, and research certainly gave no attention to the *haredim*, the strictly or ultra-orthodox Jews who because of the spiritual importance they attach to child-bearing, have enormous families, but who are not normally accessible to academic researchers. They form a rapidly-growing proportion of the Jewish community and are forecast to expand from being a smallish minority of Jews – less than 10% - to a majority as the 21st century progresses. I felt they ought to receive some research attention, and researchers in the Jewish community are now increasingly careful to make some focus on *haredim*. Widening the scope of psychology of religion research included a growing minority in the UK, Muslims. Muslim academics were very enthusiastic about expanding psychology of religion research in the Muslim community.

Also, Muslims from outside the UK came to do graduate work in this field and study of the psychology of religion in the Muslim world expanded vigorously from the late 20th century onwards, involving many Arab countries (middle-eastern and North African), Turkey and Pakistan, as well as Muslim communities in non-Muslim countries. I have particularly strong and positive memories of Ali Kose from Turkey, and Lamis Al-Solaim from Saudi (Arabia), and there were many others, Muslim, Christian and Jewish.

I set about doing research and writing articles and books that involved multi-cultural and multi-religious groups. This current monograph finalises with a focus on a development in this research which began in 2016. During the late 20th century I had the pleasure and privilege of collaborating with Stephen Frosh and Caroline Lindsey, both very eminent academically and clinically. They included in their clinical work a strong focus on the *haredi* community. They were interested in discovering the patterning of mental health among children in this community in the UK, and knowing that I had published some work on *haredim* in the UK, invited me to cooperate with them. We achieved some success in obtaining financial support for some of the work we wanted to do, though we were left feeling frustrated in not being able to continue in the directions we felt would be most interesting and useful. But there were several years of very enjoyable and useful collaboration. One day Caroline arrived at a meeting, rather breathless and excited, full of the news that she had just trained in EMDR, which she was finding to be very good. Caroline is not a person to be easily impressed. Yes, I had heard of EMDR, and even included it as a possible therapy method in my lectures covering treatments for psychological disorders. But Caroline's enthusiasm caused me to take an active step, to look into the possibility of doing the EMDR training myself. I was told that one was unlikely to be accepted for training unless one was a mental health professional, evidenced by being a fully qualified psychiatrist, clinical psychologist, or psychotherapist. As an academic, I didn't fit any of those categories. So, I was warned, send your CV to the EMDR Association, and see whether they regard you as a suitable EMDR trainee. I was happy to get a response within a couple of days, from the EMDR Academy, saying that I was acceptable for training. I enrolled for the EMDR training run by Matt Wesson and his team in the Stress and Trauma Centre. The training required some clinical work, treating a number of people suffering from the effects of trauma, and I decided to focus on women in the *haredi* community. I had a number of contacts resulting from the voluntary mental health work I had been doing in the community, and was able to complete the EMDR training successfully. I continued to treat traumatised people and one day, I encountered a past client who greeted me joyfully saying that she was delighted with the way her religious faith (*bitachon*) had recovered as a result of EMDR.

Well that left me with egg on my face. In the world of academic psychology and indeed psychiatry, I had been the noisy person clamouring for psychology, psychiatry and psychotherapy to take more notice of religion and its effects. I still am such a person. But there I was, treating people for two years for traumatisation, without a mention of religion and spirituality. The former client and I had a nice discussion, including considering the distinction between *bitochon* (religious faith or trust) and *emunah* (religious belief). Of course my EMDR training hadn't included any mention of religion or spirituality, but that's a pretty feeble excuse for someone with my interests ignoring an issue that I claim to be fundamental. Anyway, I hastily set out to find out whether my other EMDR clients – past and present – had experienced changes in religious faith. By this time I was starting to treat some clients from outside the Jewish community. Some had some religious upbringing – others, none. I found that the latter did not experience a revival or birth of faith – there was nothing to revive, and there's no obvious way in which EMDR could give birth to faith. Those who had some religious background, reported that their faith and religious activity has strengthened following EMDR. I wrote all this up in several conference and journal papers (see later for copies of these papers), including an article speculating whether faith revival is an aspect of post-traumatic growth. An exploration of religious images reported in EMDR offered an interesting route for exploring the possible role of religious and spiritual (RS) factors in faith revival and post-traumatic growth.

Much of my work on traumatisation, both clinical and academic, has been interrupted by COVID, lockdown and related disruptions. But there is plenty more to do.

SPECIAL THANKS TO

My husband, Naftali, and our dear children, Esther, Leah, Yitzi, Chana-Sora, Moshe, Rifky, Brocha, Freida, Sholi, Mendy, Zalmy, and to our children's families – to all these for their love, advice and support.

I am deeply grateful to my advisors on academic issues and matters of clinical theory and practice, and advisors on religious and spiritual matters, named in the individual papers reproduced in this volume. I will acknowledge again the continued support and blessing of the Lubavitcher Rebbe, Rabbi Menachem Mendel Schneerson.

EMDR ARTICLES AND CONFERENCE PAPERS.

These papers appeared from 2019 to 2022: as can be seen in the appendix this was alongside my other work not related to the focus here. The papers roughly show developments in my work and thinking about the main phenomenon of interest – the recovery and development of faith following trauma. There is some repetition of material: any repeated material is being used to set up a context for the argument/angle/focus of each particular paper, so I have not deleted repetitions: they are needed for contextualisation.

Conference papers were originally presented via PowerPoint slides, and the texts of these presentations have been slightly modified to make continuous prose, without altering the basic meaning. The method of referring to published articles has been modified to maintain consistency throughout.

Each paper in the series is preceded by a very short summary paragraph relating it to the development of findings and ideas in the series.

This first article describes in some detail the cases of six traumatised haredi women living in London. The article focuses on their verbal reports during EMDR, and gives an account of their reports of the improvement that they noticed following their trauma therapy.

Paper 1: Loewenthal, K.M. (2019) EMDR - Eye Movement Desensitization and Reprocessing therapy and religious faith among orthodox Jewish (*hareidi*) women. *Israel Journal of Psychiatry & Related Sciences, 56 (2), 20-27.* \ מס טיפול בתנועות עיניים ואתונה דתית\ בקרב נשים יהודיות חרדיות.
This article was previously published in the Israel Journal of Psychiatry, as cited here.

ABSTRACT

This article looks at a topic that could be of value to psychiatrists and psychologists interested in the impacts of religious cognitions on well-being: religious coping beliefs occurring spontaneously in EMDR (Eye Movement Desensitization and Reprocessing Therapy), and the reported impact of EMDR on these beliefs. The article offers brief vignettes of six *hareidi* women, focussing on changes in religious faith from trauma and trauma (EMDR) therapy. It includes transcripts from EMDR. Religious faith was shaken by trauma and generally felt to be restored in EMDR. The spontaneous appearance of experiences of religious faith was evident in EMDR transcripts as therapy proceeded. Limitations: the study involved solely women from a specific religious-cultural group. Effects need to be explored in other groups. More specific questioning before and after therapy could help to throw light on the direction of effects. The conclusions of this study are further exploration of the interactions between trauma, EMDR and religious coping beliefs would be worthwhile, in a range of cultural-religious groups.

GENERAL BACKGROUND

Trauma suffering can involve major religious struggles and doubts.

It is suggested that EMDR may be seen as freeing traumatic memory from its conditioned emotional responses, apparent in PTSD (post-traumatic stress disorder), allowing coping beliefs to induce emotional states - such as trust, faith and calmness - which had been blocked out by the terror and other negative states and behaviours characteristic of PTSD. Of course coping beliefs are not necessarily religious in content. However in cultural-religious groups in which religious coping beliefs are valued, it may be useful to be aware that EMDR may offer a relatively effective and speedy route to effective religious faith for some: those who appear to be seeking a religious trust which is eluding them, blocked by the conditioned emotional responses of fear and terror involved in PTSD.

Sample EMDR protocols and reports of the reported impact of EMDR are presented from orthodox-Jewish women.

BACKGROUND TO EMDR

Francine Shapiro (2018, p7) discovered that moving her eyes rapidly back and forth caused disturbing thoughts to abate, and when the thoughts were summoned back to mind, their negative charge was greatly reduced. Aware the eye movements played an important role in higher cortical processes,

Shapiro began to experiment with the effects of rapid back and forth eye movements on disturbing memories. Eye-movement desensitisation was applied successfully to individuals who had suffered significant traumata: rape victims and combat veterans. Techniques have been in a rapid process of development, and EMDR is now practised worldwide to address a range of clinical problems, particularly PTSD, anxiety and depression (Logie, 2014; Shapiro, 2018). It is recommended by the World Health Organization (2013) and by government mental health institutions (e.g. The UK National Institute for Health and Clinical Excellence, 2005). Volunteer organisations recruit EMDR practitioners to assist in disadvantaged communities struck by trauma.

The main stages of EMDR involve taking details of the client's current circumstances, background and stress history, developing with clients a (psychological, imaginative) "safe place" in which retreat may be sought at times of stress in the treatment or otherwise, and assessing whether the client is most comfortable with eye movements or with alternative forms of bilateral stimulation (alternate clicks in each ear, tapping on a surface towards each side of the client). Assessments of aspects of the trauma are carried out: the client is asked to envisage an image which represents the worst part of the incident/trauma. The client indicates the most salient negative self-belief brought up by the image, the most salient positive self-belief the client would like to have now, the current applicability of the positive self-belief (VoC: Validity of Cognition, rated on a 1-7 scale), the emotions felt when the image and negative self-belief are summoned now, and how disturbing the image and negative self-belief feel now (rated on a 0-10 scale), and bodily sensations experienced - if any, which and where? The most frequently-used measure is the 0-10 rating of disturbance/distress, often abbreviated as SUDS (Subjective Units of Distress). The therapist asks the clients to summon the image and then to follow the side-to-side movements (which may be of light, or sound, or of the therapist's hand). Movements are fairly rapid, approximately a second for each back and forth, and there are normally about 24 bilateral movements in a set. The client is encouraged to notice what comes to mind during each set, no matter what it is, and offer a brief report after each set. The awareness being encouraged is basically a state of mindfulness, and clients may be surprised, intrigued and sometimes amused by what comes to mind. It is usually noticeable that after a number of sets, the reported inner experiences have become less negative, more neutral or even positive. When the client reports two or three consecutively neutral or positive states, the therapist can request a Subjective Unit of Distress (SUDS) rating. The aim is that this should reduce to zero or near-zero. The therapist then assists with the installation of the positive self-belief, using bilateral stimulation, checking that this is now seen as completely applicable (a rating of 7). The therapist also checks that bodily tensions are gone when the clients recalls the trauma. With complex traumata, or clients who are troubled by several traumata, it is often necessary to repeat this core treatment.

Clients are normally relieved and pleased that their fears and tensions have been relieved, and are likely to express gratitude and pleasure that they are no longer troubled by intrusive memories and thoughts, dreams, sleep problems, anxieties, panic attacks, or other stress/PTSD symptoms.

EMDR has been a suggested treatment for a wide range of disorders, including depression, anxiety, OCD, eating disorders and others, and may be effective for any psychological disorder that can be traced to trauma

(Capeccani et al, 2013; Logie, 2014; Horst et al, 2017; Shapiro, 2018). More well-controlled research is needed.

The understanding and possibly the effectiveness of EMDR may be enhanced by the appearance of the Flash Technique (FT) (Manfield et al, 2017). FT involves sustained attention to an emotionally positive object of attention (NOT the traumatic memory), plus simultaneous bilateral stimulation, plus intermittent instructions to blink. Deliberate *inattention* to the traumatic memory is now regarded as essential in FT. This is based on work suggesting the importance of enabling traumatic memory to be processed while below the level of conscious awareness, as in FT (Siegel et al, 2017). FT may produce rapid improvements but outcome studies are still under way.

In summary, then, there is reliable evidence of the effectiveness of EMDR in treating traumatized individuals suffering from PTSD. EMDR works relatively rapidly. The neural processes involved in EMDR are still under discussion and investigation. The effectiveness of EMDR for conditions other than PTSD is suggested, but still under investigation. Reports that EMDR is found to be a generally pleasant, likeable therapy still require more investigation. FT, recently introduced as supplementary to EMDR, requires further investigation.

RELIGIOUS FAITH AND DISTRESS

There are many reports of low but generally consistent associations between a wide range of measures of religiosity, and measures reflecting lower levels of distress and psychopathology (Loewenthal, 2007; Koenig et al, 2012), although some aspects of religion may be associated with negative effects.

How might these effects come about? The fundamental work of Pargament (e.g. 1997, 2002) concluded that successful religious coping with adversity is reflected in beliefs in a just, benevolent divinity, experienced as a supportive partner in coping, involvement in religious rituals and/or a search for support through religion. These findings have been observed in a number of studies (see e.g. Gall et al, 2013; Soenke et al, 2013) and in a range of cultures: better mental health outcomes were found among both Protestant Christians and Jews who saw G-d as in ultimate control, who believed that life events were ultimately all for the best, and who experienced spiritual support (Loewenthal et al, 2000). Among Hindus the belief in *karma* - rebirth to allow for the expiation of sins committed in an earlier incarnation - may help to instil hope, and a belief in a just G-d, in stressful circumstances. Hindus feel strong obligations towards their families: these obligations strongly affect (religious) coping among Hindus (Tarakeshwar, 2013). An important feature of religious coping in many religious-cultural groups is the support provided by churches in health-related behaviours, perhaps particularly among black African-Americans (Allicock et al, 2013). Islamic beliefs and practices have a strong impact on the wellbeing of Muslims; however, it has been suggested (Abu-Raiya, 2013) that measures of Islamic religiosity require further development to enable proper understanding of the effects. The inter-relations between religion and culture are complex, and this complicates the understanding of the effects of religious coping in different cultures (Loewenthal, 2013).

A further point emerging from studies of religious coping has been the observation of coping styles and beliefs associated with poor mental health (Pargament, 1998). Notably, attention has been drawn to religious "red flags" - features of coping that have been shown to reliably predict poor mental health: belief in G-d as a punishing agent is such a red flag, as is belief in G-d as indifferent.

In this paper I report on the appearance of religious coping beliefs during EMDR, as noted while practising EMDR in a religious (orthodox Jewish) community. Religion has been suggested as a useful component in EMDR when introduced by the therapist, both for Christian and Muslim clients (Goth, 2016; Abdul-Hamid & Hughes, 2015) but this appears to be the first time that religious beliefs occurring spontaneously in EMDR have been studied.

THE CLIENTS AND THEIR COMMUNITY

Clients were recruited by networking in the strictly orthodox London Jewish community, asking for volunteers who would like to try trauma therapy in which the author was training. Six volunteers proceeded with EMDR and this is reported in this paper: subsequently a number of other women have begun EMDR with the author, who is a member of the community. All participants were strictly-orthodox Jewish (*"hareidi"*) women, living in the UK, all married, and all experienced EMDR for at least one trauma.

The strictly-orthodox Jewish community in the UK is concentrated mainly in North and Northwest London, Manchester and Gateshead, with smaller pockets elsewhere. There are estimated to be about a quarter of a million Jews in the UK, of whom 16% describe themselves as (strictly) orthodox or *hareidi* (Board of Deputies of British Jews, 2018), involving strict adherence to dietary laws, laws regarding marriage, sexuality, social relationships, entertainment, and strictly religious Jewish education.

The 6 women were all from London. Mean age at the start of therapy was 29.8 years (range 22-43), the mean number of children per family was 5 (range 1-11). To protect confidentiality and anonymity, individual demographic details are not provided. As can happen with EMDR, successful treatment of the presenting trauma sometimes opened up further issues (see below).

PROCESSING RELIGIOUS FAITH IN EMDR: CLINICAL EXAMPLES

During EMDR the client is asked to notice whatever comes to mind during bilateral stimulation (BLS) and the examples that follow shortly involve clients' reports of their experiences during BLS. Initially, there are one or more sessions in which clients describe their biography, current circumstances and life events, and agree which trauma should be focused upon first. Sometimes the client did not wish or was unable to describe the trauma, in which case a suitable EMDR-related technique was used which avoided describing or, if necessary, even consciously thinking about the trauma (B2T - blind to therapist (Blore & Holmshaw, 2009), or FT - Flash Technique (Manfield et al, 2017)). Clients received preliminary training in EMDR and (all except one) completed a brief Trauma Screening Questionnaire (Brewin et al, 2002) before undertaking EMDR. Other psychometric measures were used as appropriate, such as anxiety, depression and attachment style. This paper focuses on the verbal protocols of the women who underwent EMDR and reported on their experiences during BLS. Ratings of distress (SUDS), Validity of Cognition (VoC) (positive self-belief), and reports of bodily sensations were taken before and after EMDR. Later, women reported briefly on whether and how their religious faith had been affected by EMDR.

When beginning EMDR, clients typically have a high SUDS (7 or more up to the maximum of 10) and low VoC (typically 2 or 3). When SUDS has dropped to 0, the bodily sensations/tensions have disappeared, and the VoC has risen to 7, EMDR focuses on installing/strengthening the positive self-belief.

All women said they felt they had been traumatised. The Trauma Screening Questionnaire (26) mean score was 7.2 (range 4-9) from a maximum of 12. A score of 6 is said to be likely predictor of a PTSD diagnosis, and all except one reported at least 6 PTSD symptoms (the one exception reported 5). In all cases the women said that that they felt the EMDR successfully relieved their symptoms - symptoms such as poor sleep, intrusive memories, tension, and being easily startled, had gone. Most women continued treatment, requesting further EMDR or other therapy for issues in addition to the trauma for which they had originally sought help, for example exploring childhood experiences and family relationships.

The types of events treated with EMDR were as follows (to protect confidentiality and anonymity; general features are mentioned, with no individual details):

- Childbirth and pregnancy-related: 9

- Illness related: 4

- Childhood experiences: 6

- Anticipatory anxieties: 6.

After each set of eye-movements (or other BLS) clients reported on what had come to mind. Some examples appear later in this paper. It will be seen that there is a dream-like quality to the material that is reported by the clients.

All initially offered thoughts and images relating to their trauma(ta), with initially violent and disturbing images. Early EMDR reports had little or no religious content, but, later, clients reported some religious imagery and ideation, and/or struggles with theodicy. A widespread issue was that women felt that they knew that there was divine awareness of everything, and that what happened to them was for the best no matter how difficult, but a widespread complaint that it was difficult to *feel* the trust that they wished to experience. It was suggested to clients that their trauma(ta) had induced classically conditioned autonomic responses which were not under their current conscious control, and that EMDR could obviate the conditioned responses and enable conscious control of their feelings. Indeed, the women did report that after EMDR, autonomic symptoms had disappeared, much to their relief, and the feelings of religious trust were a common consequence of EMDR.

CASE VIGNETTES

Here follow brief accounts of each client's history in relation to EMDR, giving an overview of the progress of therapy, and including the reporting of religious coping. Following these sketches, sample transcripts from EMDR sessions give a more detailed illustration of the way images and ideas emerge.

* Mrs A has had seven EMDR sessions focussing on an agonising experience involving unsympathetic and unkind medical personnel. Images reported initially in EMDR involved shouting, blood, violence, anger at medical personnel, and physical agony. Later images began to incorporate more humane and caring medical personnel. Later sessions also involved reports of images of a bird caring for the patient, scenes involving smiles and laughter, and reports of feelings of security, safety and divine protection. The initial SUDs was 10, and was has gradually reduced to 1 with a final Flash session in which SUDS was reduced to 0.

* Mrs B had a series of hospitalisations involving problems with her ability to have children. The doctors were pessimistic. Her initial SUDS was 8. In her first two EMDR sessions Mrs B reported traumatic experiences in hospital, expressed fears of recurrences of her problems, and angry complaints at the doctors. Then she began to report more positive, hopeful thoughts ("it will pass"); the second session concluded with her optimistic expectance that *Moshiach* (the Messiah) will come" (and resolve all problems). She reported a SUDS of 4 at this point, but when returning for her third session, reported SUDS had dropped to 0 since her last EMDR session. SUDS remained at 0 throughout this session, her positive cognition was reported to be totally applicable (VoC=7), and she later reported that she continued to feel calm, with SUDS remaining at 0.

* Mrs C was prone to panic attacks resulting from fears originating in adolescence about the health of her family and friends. Bad news about the health of anyone close to her would cause a resurgence of anxiety. She also reported anticipatory anxiety, and general concerns about the safety of the world. In dealing with any given issue, early in EMDR she would report tension and struggles between her tendency to imagine catastrophic health scenarios and her wish to feel convinced that all is in divine guidance. As EMDR progressed she reported with increasing frequency feelings of

calmness and religious trust: whatever is happening is under G-d's control. Mrs C's sessions are filled with theodicy: the nature of her beliefs was not in doubt, but she struggled to *feel* the strength and tranquillity resulting from these beliefs, at all times.

* Mrs D has had 27 EMDR sessions, initially focussing on a nearly-fatal health crisis of her own. This was a complex trauma, resolved to her satisfaction after 9 sessions, when she reported that her PTSD symptoms were gone and she felt much better, no longer shaky or easily-startled and sleeping well. After this she wished to continue EMDR since she was experiencing some distress associated with memories of childhood traumata, also with issues relating to significant crises with her children's health, and with anticipatory anxieties about her own and her children's future health. The remaining 18 sessions dealt with these, including one B2T (Blind to Therapist), in which the content of the trauma was not described, but the SUDS was reduced to 0.5. In general, EMDR was initially laden with alarming images from her and her children's health crises. As EMDR progressed, religious efforts were reported (saying *Tehilim* - psalms), successful use of her safe place, images of divine protection, and reports of calmness and serenity. Her anxieties re-surface readily. In her EMDR sessions, SUDS is normally reduced, but has only once reduced to 0.

* Mrs E experienced a very severe complex event too overwhelming for her to be able to recall or think about without breaking down. We agreed to attempt the flash technique (FT) whose initial development was prompted by the need for an approach to events stimulating blocking/dissociation. FT seemed strongly indicated in this case. Initially she said she wished she could have better *bitochon* (religious trust). The traumatic event was complex and although she was unable to think about it *in toto*, Mrs E was

able to carry out FT on features of the trauma. She insisted that initial SUDS was much greater than 10 for each feature. SUDS reduced to 0 for each feature and her bodily tensions were said to have gone and her *bitochon* was strengthening.

*Mrs F reported difficult - indeed horrific - experiences in childhood and adolescence, and required 11 sessions in which talking/counselling was interspersed with EMDR. Initially during EMDR she frequently reported anger, shouting and violence, and beliefs that she would deserve divine punishments. As EMDR progressed, she reported successful efforts to prevent abuse, more kindness, laughter, dancing and cheer, while violence diminished in intensity and frequency. SUDS slowly and rather unsteadily diminished, over the 11 weeks. SUDS was 2 at the end of the 10th session. In the 11th session the flash technique was introduced, with SUDS moving to 1. She reported that for the first time she had stopped blaming herself for the horrific things that had happened to her, and wished to try a break from therapy.

EXAMPLES OF EMDR TRANSCRIPTS

Example 1

This was the seventh session for this client, and the fourth involving EMDR. The session prior to this one involved EMDR, and had started with a SUDS of 10 which reduced to 5. Her initial SUDS in this session was reported as 5, having remained stable from the finish of the previous session. What follows are her reports on what came to mind in each set:

- Seeing blood everywhere. The bird cleans up. Then he gets dirty and takes a shower.

- The bird again - calls the doctor and arranged a comfortable bed and a cosy blanket.
- (several sets in which the client reported horrific violence and agonising pain, and screaming "like I was being killed". "Hard to talk about")
- The bird is trying to come in, then comes through the back window.
- The bird tries to calm me.
- People breaking me, the bird fixing me.
- Back in the hospital bed, saying *tehilim* (psalms), *Hashem* (G-d) is with me, completely surrounding me.
- Being a in a bubble of protection, being lifted out of reach.
- Up with the moon and stars. The bird comes to join (me).

There followed several sets in which the client reported pleasant activities with the baby. SUDS reduced to 2, then 1, but did not reduce further in this session. In a further session the client wished to try the flash technique, and SUDS reduced to 0.

Example 2

This transcript is from the sixth session with a client who chose to continue having EMDR for a range of concerns which opened up after her initial, presenting trauma was desensitised. Initial SUDS was 9. Here are her reports on what came to mind in each set:
- I'm so scared, stuck, why did I do this.
- I can try to take care of myself, go to hospital, make a plan, the doctors can cope...knowing you are going to die is worse than dying.
- Why does it have to be so difficult, bringing children into the world, why so life-threatening?

- Child-bearing years don't last for ever, but 10 children for example - I can't deal with that anxiety.
- If everything goes well, I'll be so grateful. So many complications.
- Several more sets with anxious thoughts, then....
- I don't *have* to be in control.
- Imagining *Hashem* (G-d) holding my hand, steering me, I could fight, or go peacefully, with calmness.
- Much calmer when my husband is there, he expects a positive outcome, he can go with the flow...if it happens, I'm prepared, and if it doesn't, I'm grateful.

At the end of this session SUDS was only slightly lowered, to 7, but she said she could "think of getting there" (i.e. calm), and her bodily symptoms were reduced from initial chest tightness, sweatiness and tummy-ache, to solely a feeling in the pit of her stomach.

Example 3

No EMDR transcript can be given here, but reports from Flash sessions are given to indicate the nature of such reports.

This client initially gave as her negative self-belief "I have not got *bitachon* (religious trust)". SUDS was 10 plus. She attempted EMDR but did not persist, and wished to attempt the Flash Technique, in which SUDS was reduced to 0. She reported changes over the sets, progressing towards feeling easier and calmer, less angry, and said that her *bitochon* was definitely improving.

Example 4.

This client was prone to recurrent anxiety/panic attacks. This session was her twentieth, and previous sessions had been mostly devoted to EMDR which she found helpful although she remained prone to recurrent panic attacks, and was anxious about feeling anxious. Initial SUDS: 5

Here are her reports on what came to mind in each set:
- Tense feelings.
- Fearful but also feeling this (fearfulness) is not justified
- On-off tension/uncomfortable feelings
- Conflicting feelings: Frightened versus world secure, comfortable
- Again conflicting feelings. Thought that I am in charge and decide which to adopt. So I felt much calmer, more secure.
- (Both) the feelings - tried again, felt better.
- Thoughts - I'm not running the world, the One Above is running the world, and whatever does happen is the best possible thing.
- Calm and relaxed
- Initial reaction to thought of trauma, in the first second, then a calm and relaxed feeling
- Calm and relaxed, though aware that negative feelings could appear - these can be useful.

I feel I have control of feelings that are part of life (i.e. immediate reactions to stress), and I can respond to them by helping (people), *davening* (praying).
Final SUDS: 1 - this client insists that she will never reach 0 SUDS because there will always be that "initial flicker". In fact in later sessions SUDS did reduce completely to 0. All bodily tensions have gone.

Example 5.

This same client working on a different source of anxiety, SUDS 5, reported:

- Big balloon, hindering my ability to feel happy and secure, they - Hey, it's just a balloon - popped.
- Hashem has given me the ability to focus on the truth, the *neshoma* (soul), not those intruding thoughts.
- Tremor, then ignored, bounced off, focussing on inside.
- (several other sets reporting control over negative thoughts, focussing on spirituality)
- Cast all worries and fears up to Hashem who is in control - he can sort things out.

Final SUDS 3.

These examples show EMDR-typical mixtures of images, ideas and feelings. Sessions show a lessening of trauma-related imagery, ideas and feelings as the session progressed. Positive imagery, ideas and feelings, sometimes with religious or spiritual features, begin to appear.

Four of the six have since finished their trauma therapy, saying that their PTSD symptoms have reduced or gone, and reporting they feel much better, sometimes "dramatically"; one client on medication was successful in coming off medication. Recently, four clients could be contacted; they were asked whether and how they felt that their religious faith and trust (*emunah* and *bitochon*) had been affected by EMDR. Improvements were reported by each:

- It's very good, has helped greatly. There has been a positive change (in *emunah* (faith) and *bitochon* (trust)) - (I now feel that) Hashem (G-d) does good things.
- (*Emunah* and *bitochon* are) definitely climbing up, for sure.
- Definite impact. My thought processes have been clarified - what's needed for *bitochon*. As *yidden* (Jews) we all have *emunah* (faith), and EMDR is an amazing process: it really reaches *emunah* and raises it.
- *Bitochon* (trust) was not much spoken of when I was a kid - I made my own.

Bitochon is to accept not being in control. I have that in my head but not (always) in my heart. *Emunah* (faith) - is the belief that *Hashem* (G-d) is in control. I know *Hashem* is powerful and I'm not. *Hashem* can make *nisyonos* (miracles) happen, and I am not in control.

DISCUSSION

The clients described in this article were all strictly orthodox married Jewish women from the community in London. They had all undergone traumatic experiences and reported PTSD symptoms.

In EMDR, there was a general pattern of therapeutic progress, uneven but unmistakable. Initially they reported frustration that although they knew, intellectually, the characteristics of religious trust, they were unable to *feel* this trust. These reports were offered spontaneously in the course of EMDR or preliminary enquiries into emotional states.

One of the best-known reports of the impact of trauma on religious faith was Allport's (1950) study of young American men who had experienced the horrors of war, with major effects on religious faith. For some, this involved a loss of faith, while for others, their struggles served to deepen their faith. Other more recent studies on combat veterans have reported a similar loss of faith, often associated with PTSD and spiritual distress resulting from the horrors of combat (Berg, 2011; Fontana et al, 2004). The issues involved in post-traumatic spiritual growth are beginning to explored in some depth (e.g.Bray, 1999; Nijdam et al, 2018).

It is suggested here that for the women observed in this study, the process of EMDR served to free the individual from the conditioned terror responses involved in traumatisation, enabling the beliefs and feelings involved in religious faith to be experienced without a stifling blanket of terror. This enables reprocessing of memory, as has been suggested by Shapiro (2018); Adaptive Information Processing is a result of EMDR, enabling more functional processing of information stored in long-term memory). Manfield et al (2017) have suggested, somewhat similarly, that FT enables memories to be reconsolidated, although Ecker (2018) suggests that the memory content itself is not reprocessed, just its "absolutely lethal status" has been unlearned.

The observations reported in this paper suggest that once traumatic memory has been desensitised, it is possible for the previously traumatic memories to be reprocessed in the light of religious faith - which had previously been ineffective. Clients' main complaints were that although they *knew* that everything is divinely controlled, they could not *feel* this. EMDR enabled *feelings of* faith and trust to develop or re-develop.

The transcripts suggest the emergence of ideas and images reflecting religious trust; it is likely that the ingredients of these ideas and images were latent, and had been consciously accessible, and the result of therapy is to enable their positive effects on affect and the traumatic memory is desensitized and reprocessed. It has been suggested that therapists might introduce religiously appropriate ideas and practices into EMDR (Goth, 2018; Abdul-Hamid & Hughes, 2015). This was not done in the therapy reported here, but it appears that EMDR can spontaneously enable the emergence and possibly the development of spirituality (Parnell, 1996).

There remain several issues.

Firstly, the women have commented on and described their religious feelings, and their new confidence in their religious trust, aroused in the aftermath of successful EMDR and the disappearance of their symptoms. However there is scope for further exploration of ways in which they feel that the quality of their faith - intellectually and/or emotionally - has changed or deepened. There is clearly a sense in which the clients described here reflected an ever-present awareness of trauma and its impact, alongside an overwhelming sense of religious trust. There is scope for explicit examination and descriptions of ways in which this differs from pre-traumatic religious feelings, the outcomes of a *hareidi* upbringing, in which adults have attempted to inculcate children with religious faith.

Secondly, it was noted that there was one exception to the general pattern of improved faith and trust, and this was Mrs F. In her case the changes in religious coping during EMDR involved the *disappearance* of *negative religious coping.* Initially Mrs F described how she was brought up to expect that G-d would punish her, whatever she did, and these negative coping beliefs were apparent in EMDR, particularly in the earlier stages. As EMDR progressed, images and ideas became more positive, and in her final session Mrs F reported that for the first time in her life she was conscious that she had stopped blaming herself for the bad things that had happened to her, implying that she was freeing herself from the belief that she deserved divine punishment. There is scope for deeper exploration of the impact of EMDR on negative religious coping.

Thirdly, the introduction of the Flash Technique (FT) into EMDR therapy is very recent. This author has invited current clients to try it, and responses have been good, sometimes enabling therapy to be completed rapidly. Some clients are now deciding in each session whether to use FT or EMDR. FT has been greeted enthusiastically by the therapists that have trained in it, but systematic research is still awaited. FT does not give rise to nearly as much verbal descriptive material as in EMDR. To examine the processing of religious trust in FT, it would be necessary to introduce specific questions about this issue. EMDR has been throwing up material on religious/spiritual issues without prompting. FT would require more proactive enquiry from the therapist.

Finally, it is noted that this paper reports on effects observed in the UK among orthodox Jewish women. Most EMDR therapy is being practised in Western countries. Other steps in the investigation of the effects described in this paper could involve trauma victims from other cultural-religious backgrounds, men as well as women. It has been noted that EMDR may help to release feelings of spirituality, and a process of spiritual unfolding

(Parnell, 1996); the observations reported in this paper may be examples of such a process, and offer details of how this process occurs in EMDR. The processes observed here may well apply in at least some groups other than those reported here.

CONCLUSION

This paper outlined the experiences of orthodox Jewish women in the UK, undergoing EMDR for traumata. It was observed that women felt unhappy and frustrated with their loss of religious trust (*bitochon*) following trauma, and it was observed that positive religious beliefs and feelings appeared to arise in the course of EMDR. In some cases the Flash Technique was used as supplementary to EMDR. It is suggested that the effect of EMDR/FT is to undo the classical conditioning which occurred in traumatisation, enabling religious cognitions in the individual's repertoire to activate and develop previously-blocked feelings of religious trust.

ACKNOWLEDGEMENTS

Thanks to the Israel Journal of Psychiatry for permission to reproduce this article, originally published in that journal as cited at the head of this paper. Rabbinic approval for my research in general and /or for specific articles reprinted here has been given by Dayan Dunner, Dayan L.Y.Raskin and by Rabbi S.Lew, and I thank each for their kind support.

Many thanks to the clients who so kindly cooperated with the procedures described here and who allowed the publication of the transcripts and other details in this article. Also many thanks to my EMDR and psychotherapy therapy supervisors - they are not responsible for the content of this article. I owe enormous gratitude for their regular support and advice while developing my skills, such as they are, in psychotherapy and EMDR: Dr Joseph Berke, John Spector, and Lois Elliott.

References (SEE LATER)

This second paper examines the recovery of faith as reported by orthodox Jews undergoing EMDR trauma therapy. There is an interesting distinction made between Bitochon (faith) and Emunah (belief). The latter was suggested to be relatively unaffected by trauma. The former is shaken and may be lost as a result of trauma, and may recover in the course of therapy and/or other post-traumatic healing.

Paper 2: Loewenthal, K.M. (2019) Trauma and therapy: The loss and recovery of faith: An enquiry into experiences. Presented to the *World Psychiatric Association*, Jerusalem, December 2, 2019.

Abstract

This paper outlines the practice of EMDR (Eye Movement Desensitisation and Reprocessing) used in trauma therapy. The paper will describe an unexpected observation: after therapy, religiously-affiliated clients – having experienced difficulty with their religious faith following trauma and prior to therapy - then spontaneously reported the recovery of their faith as EMDR progressed. Reports and experiences during therapy, and interviews following therapy are described. These observations are discussed in the context of the literature on loss of faith and post-traumatic spiritual growth. It is noted that the EMDR literature contains negligible reference to this phenomenon, which deserves more attention.

Topics

- Trauma and faith
- What is EMDR?

- How does it work?
- Loewenthal's study of chareidi clients: their reports during and after EMDR (and Flash)
- What is faith? Emunah? Bitochon?
- The experiential study?
- How is trauma seen to affect faith?
- How are the effects of therapy on faith experienced?

Trauma and faith

Allport's (1950) classic study The Individual and His Religion included careful recording of the experiences of war veterans who found their faith shaken by their traumatic experiences. Some lost their faith, others developed a more mature faith.

More recent work includes Fontana & Rosenheck (2004), who emphasised the search for meaning resulting from trauma; Peres, Moreira Almeida, Nasello & Koenig, (2007), who emphasised the role of religion and spirituality in the quest for meaning resulting from trauma; Shaw, Joseph & Linley (2005) who examined personality and other factors associated with post-traumatic growth and the deepening religion/spirituality following trauma.

The literature on trauma and faith discusses the use of religious coping in recovery and post-traumatic growth, but there is negligible mention of the return/strengthening/development of faith as a result of therapy.

What is EMDR?   *https://youtu.be/hYy2NBXkPSo*

EMDR *reduces/eliminates negative affect associated with traumatic memory, enabling reprocessing of the memory.*

8 phases – in summary

- *Taking the client's history and circumstances, establishing a "safe place", and the identifying and (where feasible) describing the trauma claimed to be causing PTSD.*
- *Ask: what picture represents the worst part of the incident/abuse?*
- *Record SUDS*, -ve and +ve feelings and self-beliefs, and bodily sensations.*
- *Sets of BLS**, client reports images, thoughts etc. that come to mind during BLS.*
- *Reduce SUDS to 0, check bodily sensations etc.*
- *Install positive self-belief.*

*SUDS rating: Subjective Units of Distress 0-10 scale
**Bilateral Stimulation, about 20 secs: eye-movements, clicks, tapping.

How does EMDR work?

When a traumatic or very negative event occurs, information processing may be incomplete, probably because strong negative feelings or dissociation interfere with information processing. This prevents the forging of connections with more adaptive information that is held in other memory networks. The memory is unprocessed, and is implicit, emotional and subcortical. It triggers the symptoms of PTSD – which are:

1. Upsetting thoughts or memories about the event that have come into your mind against your will
2. Upsetting dreams about the event

3. Acting or feeling as though the event were happening again

4. Feeling upset by reminders of the event

5. Bodily reactions (such as fast heartbeat, stomach churning, sweatiness, dizziness) when reminded of the event

6. Difficulty falling or staying asleep

7. Irritability or outbursts of anger

8. Difficulty concentrating

9. Heightened awareness of potential dangers to yourself and others

10. Being jumpy or being startled at something unexpected

(Source: Brewin et al: Brief screening instrument for PTSD. *British Journal of Psychiatry, 2002)*

Theory and neuroscience

Stickgold (2002) suggests that EMDR may replicate the naturally occurring dream-based consolidation processes via the eye movements which are common to both REM sleep and EMDR.

I note that reports of images, ideas, thoughts during BLS often have a dream-like quality E.g:

- *Words tumbling around, evil, static.*
- *Shouting and screaming*
- *A bird comes in and blows up to be bigger than a teddy bear.*

Neuroscientists (e.g. Panksepp & Biven, 2012) speculate on the involvement of the fear circuit, including the periaqueductal grey, the amygdala and the frontal lobes.

Ecker (e.g. 2018) – memory deconsolidation and reconsolidation: traumatic memory lies outside conscious control, and is implicit and consolidated subcortically. It cannot normally be unlearned or extinguished, but if activated and during the activation period (five hours), fearful expectations are disconfirmed, symptoms may be permanently erased. Ecker calls the process reconsolidation, suggesting that it may occur in several forms of trauma therapy including EMDR.

Earlier study of *hareidi* clients: their reports during and after EMDR

This earlier study (SEE Loewenthal, 2019, above) offers brief vignettes of six *hareidi* women, focussing on changes in religious faith from trauma and trauma (EMDR) therapy.

Religious faith was shaken by trauma and generally felt to be restored in EMDR.

The spontaneous appearance of experiences of religious faith was evident in (many) EMDR transcripts as therapy proceeded.

Aims of this study

To examine the experience of faith and the nature of its loss and restoration, among traumatised strictly orthodox Jews who have undergone EMDR.

What is faith? *Emunah? Bitochon?*

Definitions - NB Both terms are often translated as **faith.**

***Emunah*:** The Rambam defines emunah as the <u>knowledge</u> that *Hashem* created and continues to run all of Creation.

***Bitochon*:** Bitachon means <u>trust</u>. The Chovos HaLevavos defines bitachon as relying on *Hashem*, trusting *Hashem*. It is a sense of depending on Him to watch over and protect me.

(From **Shafier**, 2014)

This experiential study

Participants were 10 chareidi adults (8 women, 2 men) who had received EMDR from the author were approached and asked to respond to to six questions, either in a face-to-face interview by telephone, or in writing. Six agreed (5 women, 1 man): Face-to-face: 1; Writing: 2; Telephone: 3.

Prior to receiving EMDR, all scored 6 on more on the Trauma Screening Questionnaire (Brewin et al, 2002), indicating likelihood of being diagnosed with PTSD in a clinical interview); some had received a formal psychiatric PTSD diagnosis.

The **questions** were:
1. Did you find that trauma affected your bitochon and emunah?
2. Can you describe how?
3. Did you find that EMDR affected your bitochon and emunah?
4. Can you describe how?
5. What is bitochon? (What does this word mean to you in your experience?)
6. What is emunah? (What does this word mean to you in your experience?)

Analyses:

Thematic analysis/IPA (Interpretive Phenomenological Analysis)/using a grounded theory approach.

Questions 1 and 2: How is trauma seen to affect faith (*Bitochon* and *Emunah*)?

Collectively, the responses suggested
Bitochon (trust) is affected by trauma;
Emunah (knowledge) may remain untouched.

   Trauma stimulates work on the self and/or therapy, which leads to a strengthening of *bitochon* (and *emunah*).

EG: *"Trauma affected bitochon, less (effect) on Emunah"*
"Trauma makes one question ones bitochon, and re-affirm ones emunah"
"With PTSD, I didn't feel safe or calm".

Qs 3 and 4. How are the effects of therapy on faith experienced?

A particularly significant impact of trauma therapy is on *feeling.*

EG: *"EMDR helped to process everything so that what I know in my head reached my heart".*
"After EMDR – Bitochon (changed/improved) - felt safety".
"EMDR allows one to process troubled thoughts and feeling, and (it) brought clarity and comfort when bitochon is accessed. It (EMDR) helps you to bring all that you know from subconscious to conscious, and even to elevate it to a greater level of belief in Hashem's hashgocha (providence)".

Q5. What is emunah? (What does this word mean to you in your experience?)

Emunah is *knowledge* of the nature of G-d, creating and controlling everything for ultimate good. Intellectual-level activity.

EG: *"Emunah is to believe that Hashem is controlling my life and planning everything, every little detail of my life, every little detail of the whole world".*

"Emunah is belief in Hashem. Hashem is the loving creator of the world, runs it in precise detail, and takes care of us".

"Emunah is knowing that Hashem runs the world and knows what he's doing and it's somehow all good".

What is *bitochon*? What does this word mean to you in your experience?

Bitochon is primarily a feeling-level experience. Perhaps essential that it's preceded by *emunah*. It's a feeling of trust and safety no matter what.

EG: *"Bitochon is knowing I'm not in control, and feeling calm and safe with the fact the Hashem is in contro"l.*

"Bitochon is the feeling of Hashem's loving presence in your life. It is acquired as a result (on the basis) of Emunah".

"Bitachon that he (G-d) loves us, wants us to feel all the good consciously and practically no matter who we are or what were doing or where were up to".

Some conclusions

Although some clients referred to the return of *"Bitochon and Emunah"* as a single experience or process, closer questioning suggested a distinction –

Emunah is intellectual-level belief, *Bitochon* primarily involves emotions, particularly of trust, love, safety.

Some participants seemed clear that it was possible to have *emunah* – intellectual-level belief in G-d – without *bitachon*. This may lead to post-traumatic anger or despair– how can an all-powerful G-d allow this to happen?

It appears that EMDR speeded up, indeed precipitated, post-traumatic growth; this paper focussed on the development of *bitochon.*

The observations here support the claim that EMDR does indeed desensitise traumatic memory (e.g. Shapiro, 2018)– the mechanisms of the process are still somewhat mysterious, though the process itself is evident to EMDR therapists who routinely witness the transformation of psychic processes from hideous trauma-related awareness (or related defences) to neutral or pleasant states.

There is some support for Ecker et al's (e.g. 2012) contention that EMDR is one of several trauma therapies that enables traumatic memory to be reconsolidated in a non-threatening form. Content is unaltered, they claim, while emotion is permanently erased.

In this study, religious *belief (emunah)* is an important basis for the shaping the quality of feeling – religious faith and trust *(bitochon).*

This next paper examines recovery from trauma involving EMDR, in small group of people with non-religious and religious (Christian and Jewish) backgrounds. The important conclusion of this paper is that faith recovery does not occur unless there is a religious or spiritual background. There were no cases of faith springing up new in the context of recovery from trauma.

Paper 3. Loewenthal, K.M. (2021) Religion, spirituality and recovery from trauma via EMDR therapy. Paper given at the conference of the *International Association for the Psychology of Religion* **(online), August 2021.**

Religion, spirituality and recovery from trauma via EMDR therapy

This paper outlines work on faith and trauma, and describes EMDR (Eye Movement Desensitisation and Reprocessing) therapy for trauma. There is substantial literature on EMDR as swift and effective therapy, but negligible attention to religion/spirituality (R/S) in EMDR. I began receiving reports from orthodox-Jewish EMDR clients, that their faith had been strengthened by EMDR. This paper examines this phenomenon among other clients. I interviewed nine London adults, from Christian or non-religious backgrounds.

R/S thoughts, feelings and images were recorded during EMDR, alongside other thoughts and feelings.;

I noted any reported strengthening of religious faith/spirituality as EMDR progresses.

These observations are compared with those made on the Jewish sample studied earlier. Observations considered in the context of existing literature on loss of faith in trauma, and post-traumatic spiritual growth. It is suggested that EMDR work should give more attention to R/S issues.

Trauma and faith; Trauma can shake/shatter faith, and can cause questioning

Allport (1950) in *The individual and his religion* recorded the experiences of war veterans who found their faith shaken by their traumatic experiences. Some lost their faith, others developed a more mature faith.

More recently, Fontana & Rosenheck (2004), emphasised the search for meaning resulting from trauma and associated loss of faith. Peres, Moreira Almeida, Nasello & Koenig, (2007) emphasised the role of religion and spirituality in the quest for meaning following trauma. Shaw, Joseph & Linley (2005) examined personality and other factors associated with post-traumatic growth and deepening religion/spirituality following trauma.

The literature on trauma and faith discusses the use of religious coping in recovery and post-traumatic growth, but there is negligible mention of the return/strengthening/development of faith ***as a result of therapy***, though Parnell (1996) mentions some possible positive spiritual effects.

What is EMDR?

Often effective for PTSD and anxiety disorders (e.g.Arkowits & Lilienfeld, 2012). Recommended by most government health services for these conditions. Reduces/eliminates negative affect associated with traumatic memory, enabling reprocessing of the memory. The essential features are normally.

The client's history and life circumstances are elicited, and if possible a description of the troublesome trauma(ta) (see footnote).

Various relevant features of the traumatic incident/circumstances are described and rated – including SUDS (subjective units of distress, 0-10 scale), and bodily sensations.

The central feature of EMDR is BLS (bilateral stimulation) which involves eye movements, or other stimulation in which the right and left brain are alternately stimulated. The client may report the images, thoughts etc. that come to mind during BLS, but reporting is not compulsory.

BLS is repeated until SUDS reduces to 0, bodily sensations of distress gone.

How does EMDR work?

EMDR/BLS stimulates memory reprocessing…it is suggested (from neurological evidence that) traumatic /strongly negative events are incompletely processed – probably a result of interference by dissociation or high negative emotional arousal. Connections with more adaptive information in other memory networks are made following BLS.

Traumatic memory is unprocessed, implicit, emotional and subcortical, and triggers the symptoms of PTSD. EMDR/BLS desensitises, and facilitates cortical processing.

EMDR relieves the symptoms of PTSD, including somatic symptoms, and distress.

Theory and neuroscience

Stickgold (2002) suggested that EMDR may replicate the naturally occurring dream-based consolidation processes - via the eye movements which are common to both REM sleep and EMDR.

I note that reports of images, ideas, thoughts during BLS often have a dream-like quality, e.g:

"Words tumbling around, evil, static".
"I see a rose bush, a blue door"
"A bird comes in and blows up to be bigger than a teddy bear."

Neuroscientists (e.g. Panksepp & Biven, 2012) suggest involvement of the fear circuitry, including the periaqueductal grey, the amygdala and the frontal lobes.

Ecker (e.g.2018) – suggest memory deconsolidation and reconsolidation: traumatic memory lies outside conscious control, and is implicit, subcortically consolidated, cannot normally be unlearned or extinguished. However, if activated, then during the activation period in working memory (five hours), fearful expectations are disconfirmed, symptoms may be permanently erased. Ecker calls the process reconsolidation, suggesting that it may occur in several forms of trauma therapy including EMDR. *Note that no conscious processing is necessary in desensitisation.*

My experience of EMDR

I trained in EMDR 5 years ago, and have been practising continuously since qualifying, alongside my academic work. I spend 2 days a week on therapeutic work, including supervision and further training. To date I have treated 42 clients. Number of sessions per client ranges from 1-40+

Initially my clients came from the strictly orthodox Jewish community in London, via the "grapevine". COVID lockdown forced this work to stop as face-to-face therapy became unsafe, and the majority of the community do not use the internet or computers for religious reasons. At the time of writing, lockdown is still in force.

I opened a website on Psychology Today, a psychotherapy and counselling website. I have many more enquiries from this source than I can handle, and also a number of referrals from elsewhere (previous clients, the grapevine, fellow-EMDR practitioners).

Religion and spirituality (R/S) IN CLIENTS' BACKGROUNDS

In clinical psychology, psychotherapy and psychiatry until about 10 years ago, clinicians seldom elicited information about clients' religious beliefs and activity, and spirituality. These were not considered relevant to the clinician's remit.

There has been a significant swing in general clinical practice - to incorporate R/S into patient information, but this has not yet become pronounced in the EMDR literature. Question/s about R/S need to be incorporated in the EMDR background interview.

This paper considers material from 15 clients, including reference to and comparison with 6 orthodox-Jewish EMDR clients (further description of these elsewhere) (Loewenthal, 2019, 2020). This paper involves 9 clients from the wider (non-Jewish) UK community, self-referred for EMDR therapy. I have records of EMDR therapy and their responses to questions about their religious faith, spirituality, and changes relating to trauma and trauma therapy. 5 clients had a Christian upbringing, and 4 said they had no religious upbringing.

THOUGHTS/FEELINGS DURING THERAPY

In EMDR, talk is not as crucial to therapy as in normal talk therapy. However, clients are asked to give some personal history, and comments are welcomed at any other point in therapy. Also, they are normally asked to describe what came to mind during BLS, and this may generate considerable material for some clients. For some clients, R/S thoughts, feelings and events are among the material that comes up.

The amount of talk in therapy related to R/S was limited, and the proportion of clients mentioning R/S was limited to those identifying as both religious and spiritual: 3/9 clients, also 3/6 orthodox-Jewish clients.

DURING THERAPY EXAMPLES

G-d saying to me "You're a lovely person... G-d is going to help... I say Psalm 23 (The lord is my shepherd...) I talk to G-d... My trust in G-d is coming back...Thinking about G-d is very healing. (RS)

I was more religious when young. I became lazy. Since EMDR (trauma therapy) I have become more active, going to church, more religious feeling (RS)

When my grandmother died, G-d was there the whole time. After my grandmother died I stopped churchgoing, but G-d is there the whole time, I feel everything happens for a reason...I heard a gospel song (during EMDR) which I hadn't heard for years ...wanted to take the shackles off my feet so I can dance...Faith means there is more to life than what we hear or see, believing in a higher power.(RS)

Changes in R/S in response to questioning about changes in faith following EMDR

Of the nine clients from the wider community, all three identifying as RS reported a strengthening of faith. Of the three identifying as spiritual but not religious, one reported an improvement in spiritual support, one reported improved faith but in human interaction, not spiritual. The remaining individual discussed faith and spirituality but without saying that their feelings and beliefs had shifted in therapy. Of the three with no explicit R or S identity, there was discussion by two of faith and belief, but no indication of change as a result of therapy.

	RS	S	0
Change following therapy	3	2	0
No change	0	1	3

For comparison, all the 6 (strictly orthodox) Jewish clients were aware of changes in religious faith as a result of EMDR (trauma therapy). These are described more fully in Loewenthal 2019, 2020. In brief, they claimed a roughly consistent *intellectual* level of **belief** (Hebrew *emunah*) even following trauma, but the therapy increased **trust**, an *emotional* strengthening of belief (Hebrew: *bitochon*).

Clients' descriptions of changes in faith resulting from therapy

RS

- I'm getting my faith back now. EMDR led to a huge amount of processing (RS)
- Since EMDR I have felt improvement in religious feeling. I've been more active religiously (church, prayer, study) since EMDR (RS)

- I feel closer to G-d (since therapy). I feel G-d there the whole time. I feel I've been the strong one in my religion. I don't feel alone, not alone, not alone, supported and protected (RS).

S
- A dramatic change from EMDR. I began to feel supported and guided, spiritually, but I do not use the term G-d (S).
- No faith (development or change) but I believe in things that are good for the soul (for example) connect with nature (S).
- EMDR restored some faith in human interaction, but not religious (No RS before therapy). Faith is belief that there is a conscious design, a higher power controlling life even when there is no empirical proof (S).
- No change, No R or S .
- I would like to believe in spirituality but it doesn't appear to be forthcoming in real life. Faith is a kind of insanity, longing for betterment, but not realistic (0).
- No change, but complex feelings about G-d. Angry at unfairness (of life) (0)

Conclusions

Although there was relatively little reference to religion/spirituality during therapy (as seen in the therapy transcripts), the references to R/S occurred solely in clients who identify as RS.

Improvements in religious/spiritual feelings following EMDR were reported solely in clients who identify as RS or S (Fisher's exact probability, $p<.025$).

- Among RS clients the material suggested a closer, improved relationship with G-d, and/or religious feelings and activities.

- Among S clients, improvements in spirituality and human relations were reported, but no theistic experiences or changes.
- There was no evidence of clients without religious or spiritual features in their lives developing religious or spiritual awareness or growth following trauma or trauma therapy.

The numbers of clients involved in this study were **very tiny** – sufficient to give a glimpse of **themes** that might be important, and to suggest future possibilities for quantitative analysis when larger numbers of clients can be studied.

Despite differences in cultural context (Jewish/Christian/agnostic) and associated differences in terminology, there were essential similarities in post-traumatic developments.

Questions arising:

1. How does the occurrence of RS in transcripts relate to recovery/improvement in faith?

RS identity---RS in transcript:

RS identity---recovery/improvement in RS

Causality?

2. Is the recovery of faith in RS clients following EMDR a phenomenon specific to EMDR, or an(other) example of post-traumatic spiritual growth?

This paper looks at RS change in relation to more general post traumatic growth. It considers the question whether RS change is simply a feature of overall growth and improvement, and considers the causal relationships involved.

Paper 4. Loewenthal, K. (2022) Religious change and posttraumatic growth following trauma therapy: A systematic review. *Mental Health, Religion & Culture*, 25(3), 380-387.

Psychology Department: Royal Holloway, University of London; Glyndwr University, Wales; New York University in London.

Abstract

This systematic review examined the question whether positive religious/spiritual (R/S) change is facilitated by EMDR trauma therapy. The question is asked whether any such R/S change is simply a feature of overall post traumatic growth (PTG), or is it a form of change specific to EMDR? This systematic review found a number of articles showing that R/S change could follow EMDR, and also could be a feature of overall PTG. Quantitative studies are needed to discover whether and how R/S change following EMDR is independent of PTG, or related to other aspects of PTG.

Introduction

I was carrying out EMDR trauma therapy with women from the orthodox Jewish community. They were happy with the way in which their PTSD symptoms had been eliminated, and distress levels had been reduced. Then one of my clients offered some thanks on a different topic. "It's wonderful", she said, "that my *bitochon* (Hebrew for religious and trust) has come back." Other clients offered similar reports (Loewenthal, 2019), and I went on to look at the effects of EMDR trauma therapy on religious and spiritual feelings in clients from the wider (non-Jewish) community (Loewenthal 2021).

EMDR is a form of therapy shown to be effective with PTSD and probably other disorders (see Logie, 2014; Shapiro, 2018). EMDR reduces or eliminates the negative affect associated with traumatic memory, enabling reprocessing of the memory – termed Adaptive Information Processing (AIP) by Shapiro: the "frozen" traumatic memory is adaptively processed and integrated with the individual's other life memories. A central ingredient is BLS (bilateral stimulation). The right and left brains are stimulated alternately, either by moving the eyes from side to side, or by stimulating the right and left sides of the body alternately. EMDR is now recognised by the National Institute for Health and Clinical Excellence (NICE) and the World Health Organization as a treatment of choice for post-traumatic stress disorder. It appears that eye movement desensitisation and reprocessing (EMDR) has 'come of age' as a psychological therapy on a par with cognitive behavioural therapy or psychodynamic psychotherapy.

The finding that traumatised adults who had undergone trauma therapy using EMDR were likely to report an improvement in religious faith (Loewenthal, 2019) gave rise to the question whether this change in religiosity was an aspect of general post-traumatic growth (PTG), or whether other processes are involved, specific to religion and spirituality (R/S). The question could be addressed by studying post-traumatic growth and religious/spiritual change among traumatised individuals who have undergone trauma therapy.

A related question is whether effects on religious change occur following other trauma therapy.

There have been a number of studies of PTG following trauma and trauma therapy. Shaw et al (2005) reported this in a significant systematic review, and since 2005, further studies have been published e.g. Jeon et al, (2017); Nijdam et al (2018). The most widely used measure of PTG has been the posttraumatic growth inventory (PTGI) (Tedeschi & Calhoun, 1996). Individual religiosity has proved to be a predictor of PTG. However, it is important to bear in mind that religious/spiritual change is one of the features assessed in PTG. In other words, measurement of PTG and religious/spiritual change is confounded, and without assessing the non-religious aspects of PTG separately from the religious/spiritual, we cannot learn know whether and how non-religious PTG may relate to religious change. At this point it is worth noting that the PGTI assesses five factors, including R/S: Relating to others, New possibilities, Personal strength, Spiritual change, Appreciation of life.

The research questions are

- Is positive R/S change induced by EMDR?
- Is this simply a feature of overall PTG?
- If not, how does it relate to other features of PTG?

Method

Studies of specifically religious/spiritual change following EMDR are the focus of interest and the remainder of this article reviews such studies. A systematic search of Scholar Google, Pubmed (Medline) and EBSCO (APA

PSYCHARTICLES) used the following search terms: EMDR and post traumatic growth, EMDR and religious change, EMDR and religion, EMDR and spirituality and EMDR and spiritual change.

Although there has been some controversy over the definition of the term "religious", many/most studies include an assessment of religious practice such as prayer, attendance at religious gatherings, an/or simply agreement with items of religious belief. Agreement over definition of the term "spiritual" has been less definite, with some focus on the non-material and/or the soul. Pargament's definitions of spirituality (e.g. Pargament & Exline, 2022) as search for the sacred, and search for meaning.

Searches using Scholar Google and Psycharticles produced over 1,000 hits per search (8090 was the highest number), with later hits unlikely to contain fresh material on the topic of focus (which was the improvement/increase in spiritual/religious feelings and experiences following EMDR). Hence, searches were terminated after 30 hits, giving a total of 150 hits from each of Scholar Google and Psycharticles. Pubmed/Medline produced very few results, 1-8 per search but these were scrutinised along with the 150 results from each of Scholar Google and Psycharticles (EBSCO).

Results

Author	Year	Title	Participants/ sources/s of information.	Method	Summary of relevant findings
Parnell	1996	Eye movement desensitization and reprocessing(EMDR) and spiritual unfolding.	Based on author's clinical experience with EMDR clients. Some illustrative case-based material.	Observations of clients undergoing EMDR therapy.	In the end phase, clients integrate their experiences and often feel an awakening of their creativity and spirituality. EMDR leads to spiritual unfolding.
Turpin	1999	An exploration of reported transpersonal/spiritual experiences during and after movement desensitization and reprocessing (EMDR) treatment of traumatic memories	Of 50 EMDR facilitators responding to a questionnaire, 11 were interviewed in depth about transpersonal/spiritual experiences during or following EMDR.	Questionnaire sent to EMDR facilitators on transpersonal/spiritual experiences during or following EMDR: quantitative analysis however did not lead to more global statements, so 11 facilitators were interviewed in depth.	Clients were observed reporting transpersonal/spiritual experiences following EMDR. Spiritual experiences reported during and after EMDR. Spiritual experiences are experiences interpreted as sacred, often involve a sense of higher reality and a feeling of awe. Examples: presence of deceased grandparent, comforting the client. Presence of G-d.
Mayer	2013	EMDR, spirituality, and healing in children.	Clinical experience with EMDR clients. Literature review.	Clinical experience, also published sources of theoretical orientation.	The EMDR process moves the clients to a spiritual meaning-making that seems to foster more positive emotional states and adaptive behaviors. Theoretical support from theologians, religious educators and EMDR specialists is presented especially in regard to clients' self-transcendent experiences.
Dansiger	2010	The Role of Spirituality in the Etiology and Treatment of Complex Post Traumatic Stress Disorder	Literature review	Literature review focused on measurement of spirituality, and empirical studies of spiritually based interventions used in treating trauma-related disorders: mindfulness, DBT, meditation, acceptance of emotions.	Evidence that trauma has a distinct impact on spirituality, often involving spiritual crisis, possible loss of spirituality, and development of psychopathology. Spiritual experiences may occur during and after EMDR, and spiritual practices such as mindfulness and acceptance can be usefully incorporate into clinical practice. Currently the results of EMDR treatment may be seen as spiritually based, but this needs further development.
Krystal et al	2002	Transpersonal psychology, Eastern nondual philosophy, and EMDR.	Literature review	Literature review integrating transpersonal psychology and eastern non-dual philosophy with EMDR.	Clients may report mindful awareness during EMDR sessions. clients sometimes report contact with this profound awareness during a session. EMDR has a surprising and powerful contribution to make to transpersonal psychology by helping to facilitate and stabilize the experience of nondual awareness
Loewenth al	2019	EMDR-Eye Movement Desensitization and Reprocessing Therapy and Religious Faith Among Orthodox Jewish (Haredi) Women	6 orthodox Jewish women EMDR clients	Reports of religious experiences during EMDR and responses to a questionnaire/interview after EMDR	Religious faith was shaken by trauma and generally felt to be restored in EMDR, though (cognitive) belief was adhered to. Clients reported the re-appearance/strengthening of religious faith, in EMDR transcripts as therapy proceeded, and in response to questioning after EMDR.
Loewenth al	2021	Religion, spirituality and recovery from trauma via EMDR therapy.	9 adult EMDR clients, 3 Christian, 3 spiritual, 3 non-believers.	Reports of religious experiences during EMDR and responses to a questionnaire/interview after EMDR	Strengthening/return of religious faith was experienced by clients identified as religious. Spiritual clients reported some spiritual experiences. Those identified as non-believers did not report any religious or spiritual experiences. Religious/spiritual identity and knowledge may be important in providing a framework for religious/spiritual experiences in EMDR.

Parnell	2013	Attachment-focused EMDR: Healing relational trauma	Based on author's clinical experience with EMDR clients. Some illustrative case-based material.	Observations of clients undergoing attachment-focussed EMDR therapy	In the end phase of EMDR, creativity, spirituality, and integration are the focus, with less EMDR and more talking. Questions such as "Who am I?" and "What do I want to do with my life?" arise and need to be addressed.
Siegel	2018	EMDR as a transpersonal therapy: A trauma-focused approach to awakening consciousness	2 case histories.	Using the case history material, discusses how features of transpersonal psychology might be integrated with EMDR to facilitate rich spiritual experiences.	During EMDR one client entered deep into a meditative state, different than the standard protocol. This state change fostered an expanded awareness of safety within a larger cosmic whole, and brought great joy to her experience. The other client experienced flowers growing from his head. The therapist integrated these experiences with mindful awareness, attunement and resonance, integrating EMDR induced experiences with transpersonal experiences.
Jeon et al	2017	Eye movement desensitization and reprocessing to facilitate posttraumatic growth: A prospective clinical pilot study on ferry disaster survivors	10 survivors of a major marine disaster near S Korea in 2014.	Eight EMDR sessions were administered by a psychiatrist at two-week intervals over a period of five months. Post-Traumatic Growth Inventory (PTGI), Stress-Related Growth Scale (SRGS), Clinician-Administered PTSD Scale (CAPS), and Connor-Davidson Resilience Scale (CD-RISC) were measured before treatment, after sessions 4 and 8, and three months after treatment completion.	EMDR therapy using the standard protocol for trauma processing facilitated the development of post-traumatic growth, and reduction in PTSD symptoms was associated with post-traumatic and stress-related growth.
Nijdam et al	2018	Turning wounds into wisdom: Posttraumatic growth over the course of two types of trauma-focused psychotherapy in patients with PTSD	116 outpatients diagnosed with PTSD. RCT (randomised control trial) comparing two forms of trauma therapy (EMDR and Brief Eclectic Psychotherapy for PTSD - BEP)	Self-reported and physician-rated posttraumatic growth scores were assessed pre-and post treatment. PTSD severity was measured weekly.	Posttraumatic growth scores significantly increased after trauma-focused psychotherapy, as well as scores in the subdomains personal strength, new possibilities, relating to others, and appreciation of life. No differences in this respect between the two forms of therapy. Posttraumatic growth was significantly relation to improvement in PTSD (ie decline in PTSD symptoms)
Blore	2012	An interpretative phenomenological analysis (IPA) investigation of positive psychological change (PPC), including post traumatic growth (PTG)	12 participants who had experienced a (major0 RTA.	Semi-structured interviews, IPA.	As well as negative psychological impacts, there was positive psychological growth. FLU (figurative language use) seemed to hallmark expansion of memory networks as part of a general maturation process post-RTA. Furthermore, there was evidence that participants were incorporating their traumatic experiences via FLU into the rebuilding of their assumptive worlds. These analyses contribute to the understanding of AIP (adaptive information processing which is a feature of EMDR) via posttraumatic growth

Religious change and EMDR

Table 1. The effects of EMDR on R/S (Religion/Spirituality) and PTG (Posttraumatic Growth): earlier studies summarised.

The primary research question is whether religion/spirituality has been specifically affected by EMDR. The studies identified proved to be mainly qualitative, offering reports by therapists and clients; there appear to be no studies involving quantitative measurement of before and after religiosity Although the final three studies focused on PTG as an outcome, the authors and participants gave some note to the religious/spiritual feelings experienced post-traumatically. Two of these three studies were the only quantitative studies that came up in this review. Note the first eight studies, all report and emphasise religious/spiritual posttraumatic change following EMDR, but none of these studies are quantitative.

We can draw several conclusions from Table 1:

- Positive R/S change can certainly result from EMDR.
- PTG is also a result, and the current state of information does not permit us to analyse whether positive R/S change is part of a general PTG, or whether the different features of PTG may influence each other – for example might an improvement in affectional bonds help to improve R/S feelings, and/or vice versa.
- It would be helpful if the different components of PTG were analysed separately and their inter-relationships examined.
- Pre- and post-therapy measures of R/S are needed. Although the PTGI gives a measure of R/S, this is based on only two items, and more subtle and discriminating measures would be worthwhile.
- Only one study comparing EMDR to other trauma therapy was reported (Nijdam et al). This showed comparable effects of the two forms of therapy studied on PTG. R/S effects were not examined separately. Insofar as it goes this suggests that compared to other

trauma therapy, there may be no unique effects of EMDR on PTG and its components, but a great deal more data are required.

Additionally, it can be noted that Loewenthal (2021) reported that R/S change following EMDR was reported only by those with a prior R/S identity/history. Participants without prior R/S beliefs reported no R/S changes at all. The numbers in this study were very small but the effects were statistically significant. If this finding remains consistent, it may indicate an important factor explaining the widespread report that prior religiosity is a predictor of PTG. The effect would be at least partly because R/S is included in the measurement of PTG. But it is consistent with the view that a religious/spiritual belief framework will be important in shaping reactions to trauma (Loewenthal et al, 2000).

Further investigation could include the question whether R/S changes relate to specific features of PTG. More rigour in the definition and assessment of R/S would be helpful.

Conclusions

Positive R/S change as a result of EMDR has been reported a number of times, but reports are usually solely observational and require greater rigour and structure in the assessment of R/S and its changes.

Measures of PTG include some assessment of R/S and it is possible that existing data may lend itself to examination of changes in the separate features of PTG and their inter-relations, including the relations of R/S to other features of PTG.

Comparison could be made of the effects of EMDR with the effects of other forms of therapy on PTG and R/S.

Acknowledgements

Grateful acknowledgements to New York University in London for the award of a Distinguished Research Fellowship facilitating the preparation of this paper.

Very many thanks to the EMDR users whose experiences and reflections led to this paper, and which have been have been so interesting and important to me.

This paper is the final one in this collection, though hopefully not the final one on the topic addressed: ie the post-traumatic recovery of faith. The paper was part of a fascinating symposium organised by Tasia Scrutton at Leeds University, based on the idea that some experiences may be both mystical and psychopathological. I had become very interested in the dream-like, often mystical quality of the experiences sometimes reported by clients engaged in EMDR. This paper examines these experiences, considering the question of whether they have any psychopathological qualities, and considering their role in clients' recovery of religious faith following trauma therapy.

Paper 5. Religious experiences reported during trauma therapy
A paper given at the Psychopathology and Religious Experience Symposium, Saltaire/Leeds University, April 2022

This paper outlines the practice of EMDR) Eye Movement Desensitisation and Reprocessing (used in trauma therapy. The original basic form of EMDR involved the patient/client reporting what thoughts and images came to mind while they were undergoing bilateral stimulation, of the right and left brain hemispheres alternately. These reports can often be seen as having a dream-like quality.

I examined reports from 50 clients and found a small number of reported religious experiences. These experiences are compared to dream, daydream and psychotic experiences. The question is considered whether these verbal reports are therapeutically necessary (as in psychotherapy). The relationship of religious experiences to post traumatic growth and religious change is also examined

Introduction: EMDR trauma therapy

 https//:youtu.be/hYy2NBXkPSo

EMDR trauma therapy reduces/eliminates negative affect associated with traumatic memory ,enabling reprocessing of the memory. There are eight phases – in summary

- Taking the client's history and circumstances
- Establishing a "safe place" (mental refuge)
- Where feasible, describing the trauma claimed to be causing PTSD
- Ask :what picture represents (the worst part of) the incident/abuse ?
- Record SUDS (Subjective Units of Distress) - ,* -ve and+ ve feelings and self-beliefs ,and bodily sensations .
- The most lengthy stage in EMDR: Sets of (Bilateral Stimulation) BLS ,**client normally reports images ,thoughts etc .that come to mind during BLS***.
- When SUDS reduced to 0 , check bodily sensations etc.
- Install positive self-belief/s.

SUDS rating, Subjective Units of Distress, 0-10 scale

**Bilateral Stimulation ,about 20 secs :eye-movements ,clicks ,tapping.*

***It is NOT necessary for the client to describe or even to be aware of the trauma content, indeed the distress level may be too great to allow articulation of the trauma memory .EMDR can still be carried out ,for instance using B2T) Blind to Therapist ,(or Flash .In the latter ,the client actively focuses attention away from the trauma memory onto a PEF)Positive Engaging Focus.

EMDR was first developed by Francine Shapiro (eg. Shapiro, 2018; de Jongh et al, 2020). Has Spread very widely and rapidly.

Effectiveness well-established, especially for PTSD resulting from a single trauma (eg. Valiente-Gomez et al, 2017). Recommended by most regulatory bodies in the UK, Europe, North and South America and the Middle East including:

- The World Health Organization (2013)
- The American Psychiatric Association (2004 & 2009);
- The US Department of Defence/Veterans Affairs (2004 & 2010), and
- The International Society for Traumatic Stress Studies (2000 & 2008).

UK NICE (National Institute for Clinical Excellence: recommendations for the NHS) (2005)

PTSD (Post-Traumatic Stress Disorder)

When a traumatic or very negative event occurs ,information processing may be incomplete, probably because strong negative feelings or dissociation interfere with information processing .This prevents the forging of connections with more adaptive information that is held in other memory networks .The memory is unprocessed and is implicit , emotional and subcortical .It triggers the symptoms of PTSD – which are:

- Upsetting thoughts or memories about the event that have come into your mind against your will

- Upsetting dreams about the event

. Acting or feeling as though the event were happening again .

- Feeling upset by reminders of the event

- Bodily reactions) such as fast heartbeat ,stomach churning ,sweatiness , dizziness (when reminded of the event

- Difficulty falling or staying asleep

- Irritability or outbursts of anger

- Difficulty concentrating

- Heightened awareness of potential dangers to yourself and others.

- Being jumpy or being startled at something unexpected

(Source :Brewin et al :Brief screening instrument for PTSD . *British Journal of Psychiatry.2002)*

Some of the processes involved in traumatisation include Stickgold's suggestion (2002) that EMDR may replicate the naturally occurring dream-based consolidation processes via the eye movements, which are common to both REM sleep and EMDR.

I note that reports of images ,ideas ,thoughts during BLS often have a dream-like quality, for example:

- *"Words tumbling around, evil, static".*
- *"Shouting and screaming".*
- *"A bird comes in and blows up to be bigger than a teddy bear".*

Ecker (2018) argues that traumatic memory lies outside conscious control, and is implicit and consolidated subcortically. It cannot normally be unlearned or extinguished, but if activated, then during the activation period (about five hours), fearful expectations are disconfirmed, and symptoms may be permanently erased .Ecker calls the process reconsolidation, suggesting that it may occur in several forms of trauma therapy including EMDR.

Neuroscientists such as Stickgold (2002) suggest the weakening of the involvement of the hippocampus and the amygdala (midbrain structures) with the traumatic memory during EMDR, and increase in frontal lobe (forebrain) involvement.

It appears that EMDR speeded up, indeed precipitated, post-traumatic growth; this paper focussed on the development of religious faith in the context of the study of post-traumatic growth.

The observations here support the claim that EMDR does indeed desensitise traumatic memory .(E.g.Shapiro, 2018). The mechanisms of the process are still somewhat mysterious , though the process itself is evident to EMDR therapists who routinely witness the transformation of psychic processes from hideous trauma-related awareness) or related defences (to neutral or pleasant states .

There is some support for Ecker's contention that EMDR is one of several trauma therapies that enables traumatic memory to be reconsolidated in a non-threatening form. Content is unaltered ,while emotion is permanently erased.

Some religious Jewish clients suggested - religious *belief* (*emunah*) is intellectual and not so affected by trauma. Religious faith and trust (*bitachon*) (emotional) are damaged by trauma, may be restored in EMDR.

Some of my academic history.

Post doctorally, I did full-time academic, teaching and research, 1967-2007. My main interests were the psychology of religion (religion and mental health), research methods, psychodynamic therapy. I also did some voluntary work, mainly relating to mental health.

Post-retirement I continued with some teaching and research. I was more involved with voluntary work, especially Chizuk in the orthodox-Jewish community, and the National Spirituality and Mental Health Foundation nationally. I qualified in EMDR in2017 , and practise this part-time. I have treated over 50 clients for PTSD, mainly using EMDR ,sometimes including EMDR-related methods, specifically Flash and B2T.
Among my recent publications, I include 3 recent conference presentations and 2 articles in peer-reviewed journals on my EMDR work

Examples of sets and images

To give a fuller illustration of the sequence and range of ideas and images that come to mind in EMDR, four examples of EMDR **sets** are shown, followed by examples of **single experiences/images.** To help preserve confidentiality/anonymity, demographic features have not been stated.

Within each set, we can see that earlier reports reflecting a high level of distress, often clearly relating to the client's trauma; later in the set, more positive feelings and thoughts appear, again characteristic of the processes involved in EMDR. Reports of religious/spiritual/mystical (RSM) ideas and feelings may be made (by some clients). These normally appear alongside the more positive reports/images/feelings.

EXAMPLE A

- Seeing blood everywhere. The bird cleans up. Then he gets dirty and takes a shower.

- The bird again – calls the doctor and arranged a comfortable bed and a cosy blanket.

- (Several sets in which the client reported horrific violence and agonizing pain, and screaming "like I was being killed." "Hard to talk about.")

- The bird is trying to come in, then comes through the back window.

- The bird tries to calm me.

- People breaking me, the bird fixing me.

- Back in the hospital bed, saying Tehilim (Psalms), Hashem (G-d) is with me, completely surrounding me.

- Being a in a bubble of protection, being lifted out of reach.

- Up with the moon and stars. The bird comes to join (me).
- Tense feelings.

Example B

- Fearful but also feeling this (fearfulness) is not justified

- On-off tension/uncomfortable feelings

- Conflicting feelings: Frightened versus world secure, comfortable

- Again conflicting feelings. Thought that I am in charge and decide which to adopt. So I felt much calmer, more secure.

- (Both) the feelings - tried again, felt better.

- Thoughts - I'm not running the world, the One Above is running the world, and whatever does happen is the best possible thing.

- Calm and relaxed

- Initial reaction to thought of trauma, in the first second, then a calm and relaxed feeling

- Calm and relaxed, though aware that negative feelings could appear - these can be useful.

- I feel I have control of feelings that are part of life (i.e. immediate reactions to stress), and I can respond to them by helping (people), *davening* (praying).

Example C

-memory of previous therapy

- Remember movie David Lynch, (seen) in London

- Hope that I will be able to find a passion in my life

- Imagine what it's like to have a family, someone almost an extension of self

-Thinking about autumn, beautiful weather

-image of the river – Thames

-Image of a friend, asked me to ask you if you do hypnotherapy

-thinking of the pictures on the wall, nice to see all those people (in the pictures)

- vague thoughts about (my) own family – not having that kind of love, connection

-make an effort to make that connection with my friends – doesn't feel enough

-mountain and horses

-trying to force a positive image

-things in the room

-remembered an animal skin in the room of previous therapist

-just a feeling of loneliness (shakes head)

-Sound of wind outside

- (shakes head) nothing

-just a word – mother

Example D

- wondering if they have any idea what they put me through

- struggling to understand, the situation with my uncle (who abused her sexually), someone came in and went out, probably my mother, so hard to understand, she did drink a lot

- I feel I've been in a prison that I didn't know I was in – now there's a light at the end of the tunnel

- a few weeks ago I was doing all these personal development things, but not sure I was getting anywhere. Now I feel hopeful.

-a gospel song: take the shackles off my feet so I can dance – is that coincidence, I haven't heard it for years.

- the same song

- singing again. How much I underestimated my relationship with G-d. A different song: the sun rises, the sun sets. G-d is real. I've always believed in G-d - now stronger than ever before.

- it's ok to let go, for the SUDS (distress level) to be zero.

Examples of single experiences reported during EMDR

The typology I used was supported by following a procedure recommended by Elliott et al (1999): an academic colleague was asked to place the sample statements in the appropriate category, then if necessary, adjustments were made.

The initial typology followed that used in categorising the experiences emerging in EMDR: Emotionally Negative, Neutral, Positive. A further category used here was: Religious/spiritual.

Since religious experiences were relatively rare, and they are the focus of interest here, all are reported. Only a sample of the other experiences are reported.

Negative reported experiences (each from different session with different client)

- Feeling how alone I was
- Memory of him doing it (CSA)
- School teacher, unfair, picking on me
- When grandmother died, I cried every night for a year, in bed. Was not allowed to cry, mother saw it as a sign of weakness.
- At a dinner party, phone call from wife (now ex), called me horrible names, cheating scumbag, everyone staring at me
- Sitting on the floor, kids around me, spitting at me
- Lots of blackness, aloneness, vulnerability, unsupported, left alone, lost, sad, grief, huge chain of lostness.
- They were in a panic asking where my husband is, feeling I'm going to die.
- (He) tried to touch me ...(I) didn't let (him), then he tickled me roughly, angrily.
- Ambulances, a whole of ambulances and new cars.

Neutral experiences (each from a different client)

- The walk, coming to see you (therapist)
- Having dinner round the kitchen table, brother kicking a football
- Pictures on the wall (of the therapy room)
- Thinking of talking to a client in a grocery shop
- Child on a scooter crossing the road
- Nothing came to my mind
- I thought about a car boot sale I wanted to go to, trying to remember which day.

- Just thinking about work, how many emails I've got to do.

Positive experiences (each from a different client)

- My nieces and nephews visiting, planning games, I love children
- Remembering grandmother, many happy memories, I loved her.
- Memory of walking to playgroup, dressed up as Peter Pan, . Being carried on Mum's back.
- Thinking about how far I've come
- A rising feeling of power, wanting to stand up to it
- Hard to describe, a kind of feeling of belonging.
- Plans for this weekend - to see friends who want to see me.
- Tickling my baby, laughing.
- Feel as if I'm being put at my ease, a rare occurrence these days.
- I am who I am. Everything else (anxiety) has drifted away.
- Calm and relaxed

Religious/Spiritual experiences (Jewish clients)

- Hashem is the one controlling the world so no reason to be afraid
- Love from Hashem transforms pain.
- Dancing. Realising that Hashem is a loving father. The world is a beautiful place. We have to find beauty – (it's) hidden – (there are) flashes of Hashem's love and intervention. If we seek Hashem we find him.
- When we are davening (praying), trying to concentrate (whole school davens together)
- Chanuka – parties – lighting menorah, father and brother.
- Several images/scenes during BLS involving white bird protecting client against malignant medical personnel: see example A above.

- Thinking about davening – everything should be good – Hashem knows what's best, but hope He agrees with me.
- My spiritual self is my real self...it's intrinsic, in myself, unbreakable. I am valuable, precious, valid.
- Remembered visiting the Rebbe as a child (with my family). The Rebbe offered us sweets, held out his hand with the sweets, purple and orange. The Rebbe's presence filled the whole room. The purple looks exciting, the orange tastes nicer, our parents were impatient (for me to choose). The Rebbe is telling me I am able to make choices in my life. The Rebbe is standing behind me, helping me make choices (client crying).
- Mystical, spiritual, unravelling, a light is there, there's an opening.
- Being in a bubble of protection - being lifted out of reach.
- Up with the moons and stars, singing, (a) bird comes to join (me).

Imagining *Hashem* (G-d) holding my hand, steering me... peacefully, with calmness.

Religious/Spiritual (from non-Jewish clients, all here had Christian backgrounds)

- Felt improvement in religious engagement, more active involvement in church.
- Said to myself, let G-d do whatever and just let go.
- A gospel song: take the shackles off my feet so I can dance – is that coincidence, I haven't heard it for years…
- Nothing clear, really random memories, my boyfriend in secondary school, the church I went to.
- Singing again. How much I underestimated my relationship with G-d.

- The sun rises, the sun sets. G-d is real. I've always believed in G-d - now stronger than ever before.

COMMENTS

Religious experiences in EMDR were relatively rare: 19 such experiences were found in the often-voluminous records of 50 clients. The majority were reported by Jewish clients, who mainly came from the strictly orthodox Jewish community. The remaining clients were mainly from a website offering psychotherapy, often with no or minimal religious background, plus a few grapevine referrals.

Improvement in religious faith/spirituality was reported spontaneously by some clients. Following this reporting, I started to question all clients about changes in religious faith/spirituality, following EMDR, and their prior religiosity. All those with at least some religious background reported a change (improvement) in faith and/or practice. Those without a religious background reported no such changes.

Several questions arise. Are the reported experiences dream-like? Do the reported experiences have a psychotic quality? Psychosis has been compared to a dream (nightmare) from which one cannot awake. How do the reported EMDR experiences compare with daydreams? Daydreams often involve wishful thinking, and are much more readily controlled than dreams. Experiences during EMDR are subject to some level of control, and clients may request advice on how to occupy their minds during BLS. If they ask, they are advised to let their minds roam freely. This follows pre-BLS focus on the identified trauma-related target. (Clients opting for Flash select a PEF (pleasant engaging focus), and therefore the BLS experiences are nor spontaneously arising images and feelings, so they do not report BLS experiences in the same way as other clients.

One aspect of observations arising from experiences in EMDR involves the issue of the controllability and pleasantness of experiences. Speculatively,

On controllability:

Daydreams > EMDR experiences>psychotic experiences and dreams

On pleasantness:

Daydreams > dreams> EMDR experiences>psychotic experiences and nightmares.

An important issue is what are the crucial components of EMDR (resulting in clinical improvements)? What role is played by verbal reports in the desensitisation (healing) processes in EMDR? There is no evidence that experiences during BLS have to be reported/experienced in order for EMDR to be effective. Notably, "Blind to therapist" (B2T) (Blore et al, 2013) and the Flash techniques (Manfield et al, 2017) are forms of EMDR that do not require reporting of experiences during BLS, and both are reported effective. Flash actively encourages focus on a positive image (Positive Engaging Focus: PEF, *not* related to the trauma) during BLS ie. the client practising Flash could not have the (possibly) dream-like experiences discussed in this paper, as their attention is engaged elsewhere, on the PEF.

BLS (bilateral stimulation) maybe the essential component of therapy, and eye movements may be important (eg. Jeffries & Davies, 2013) …but other forms of BLS do not involve eye movement, and the therapy is still effective (see next slide). This is a puzzle if holding to the view that eye movements in EMDR are effective because similar to the eye movements in REM (dreaming) sleep.

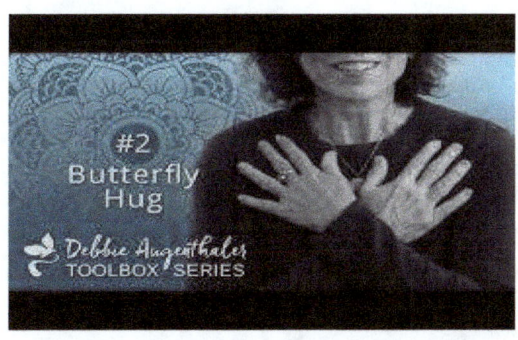

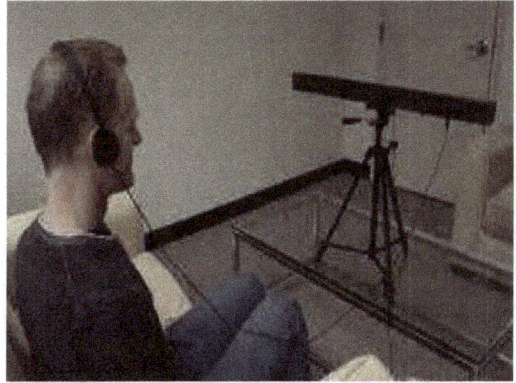

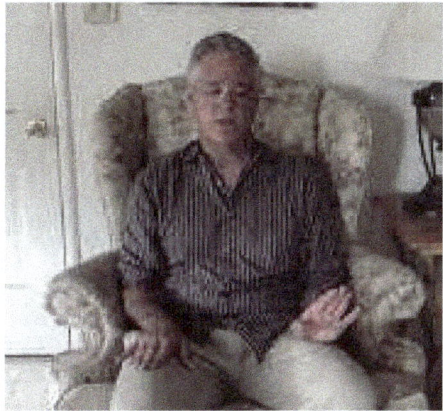

Other forms of BLS not involving eye movement, shown above are: Butterfly hug, clicking in alternate ears, tapping alternate knees/thighs.

It is significant to note that clients who reported religious experiences during BLS were more likely to report changes (improvements) in faith/spirituality, compared to those who did not report religious experiences. But causality is unclear.

I note that there have been some (rather rare) published reports of spiritual/religious growth and experiences in EMDR, though verbatim reports have not been examined/reported in detail (Parnell, 1996; Peres et al, 2006, Shaw et al, 2005).

CONCLUSION

The relationships of EMDR & related therapies to post traumatic growth (PTG) and religious change deserve further study. The nature and role of religious experiences in EMDR deserve further study. Though not frequent, they were often seen as important.

FINAL SECTION OF MONOGRAPH: CONCLUSIONS AND QUESTIONS.

So far – and in spite of the relatively small numbers of clients seen – I feel pretty confident that for clients with any feeling for religion/spirituality, EMDR is likely to touch this aspect of human feeling. Particularly, I suspect that religious counsellors, clergy and pastors etc may find that EMDR could be a route to religious consolation for those who are unhappy that their faith has been damaged or destroyed by trauma. So one possible positive suggestion arising from this area of work is the application of EMDR and probably other forms of trauma therapy in helping people unhappy about their loss of faith as a result of traumatic damage.

Another important conclusion is the result of the smallness of the numbers of people seen, and a result of their demography. We need to know whether the effects we have would hold up in larger numbers of people, and in other groups – Muslims for example, and nonreligious Jews.

Finally, I feel there are important theoretical questions that might be addressed, particularly in connection with the nature of psychosis, and of religious experience, and of dreams. Tasia Scrutton has been vigorously pushing for enquiries into the nature of psychosis, particularly pursuing the argument that it is possibly for some experiences to be both religious and psychotic. I feel that further work on the nature of dreams could be important in this connection. It has been suggested that EMDR may stimulate the same kind of brain processes that occur in dreams. We now know that this cannot simply be the result of eye movements as such, since EMDR now often uses methods of bilateral stimulation which do not involve eye movement. Nevertheless, the bilateral stimulation feature of EMDR may stimulate the dream-like features of the reports made by those undergoing this therapy.

The suggestion that psychotic experiences have a dream-like quality needs further investigation in connection with all this.

So I would like to suggest make three definite suggestions:

1. **That psychotherapy and particularly trauma therapy, and perhaps particularly EMDR, might be suggested for those who find their trauma-related religious doubts oppressive.**

2. **That we need to extend research into the question whether trauma therapy really does facilitate the restoration or redevelopment of religious faith, among groups of people for whom this phenomenon had yet to be investigated.**

3. **Finally I believe there is important work to be done on the nature and inter-relationship between dreams, psychotic experiences, religious experiences and the experiences that can occur in trauma therapy.**

REFERENCES

Allicock, M., Resnicow, K., Hooten, E.G., Campbell, M.K. (2013) Faith and health behaviour: The role of the African American church in health promotion and disease prevention. In Pargament, K.I., Exline, K., Jones, J., et al, editors. *APA Handbook of psychology, religion and spirituality.* Washington, D.C.: American Psychological Association, 439-459.

Allport, G.W. (1950) *The individual and his religion.* New York, N.Y.: Macmillan.

Abdul-Hamid, W.K., Hughes, J.H. (2015) Integration of religion and spirituality into trauma psychotherapy: An example in Sufism? *Journal of EMDR Practice and Research,* 9, 150-156.

Abu-Raiya, H. (2013) The psychology of Islam: Current empirically-based knowledge, potential challenges and directions for future research. In Pargament, K.I., Exline, K., Jones, J., et al, editors. *APA Handbook of psychology, religion and spirituality.* Washington, D.C.: American Psychological Association, 681-695.

Allicock African American church in health promotion and disease prevention. In Pargament, K.I., Exline, K., Jones, J., et al, editors. *APA Handbook of psychology, religion and spirituality.* Washington, D.C.: American Psychological Association, 439-459.

Arkowitz, H. & Lilienfeld, S.O. (2012) *"EMDR: Taking a Closer Look". Scientific American Special Editions 17, 4s, 10-11 (August 2012).* doi:10.1038/scientificamerican1207-10sp

Berg, G. (2011) The relationship between spiritu*al distress, PTSD and depression in Vietnam combat veterans. Journal of Pastoral Care and Counselling,* 65, 1-11.

Brewin, C.R., Rose, S., Andrews, B., et al. (2002) Brief screening instrument for post-traumatic stress disorder. *British Journal of Psychiatry,* 181, 158-162. https://doi.org/10.1192/bjp.181.2.158

Blore, D. (2012) *An interpretative phenomenological analysis (IPA) investigation of positive psychological change (PPC), including post traumatic growth (PTG).* Birmingham, UK. University of Birmingham PhD thesis.

Blore, D. & Holmshaw, M. (2009) EMDR "blind to therapist protocol". In Luber, M, editor. *Eye movement desensitization and reprocessing (EMDR) scripted protocols: Basics and special situations.* New York, N.Y.: Springer, 233-240.

Board of Deputies of British Jews. *Jews in numbers.* https://www.bod.org.uk/jewish-facts-info/jews-in-numbers/ (accessed 06.7.18).

Bray, P. (2016) A broader framework for exploring the influence of spiritual experience in the wake of stressful life events: examining connections between posttraumatic growth and psycho-spiritual transformation. *Mental Health Religion and Culture,* 13, 293-308. https://doi.org/10.1080/136746709033671999.

Capezzani, L, Ostacoli, L, Cavallo, M., et al. (2013) EMDR and CBT for cancer patients: Comparative study of effects on PTSD, anxiety, and depression. *Journal of EMDR Practice and Research*, 7, 134-143. doi: https://doi.org/10.1891/1933-3196.7.3.134

Dansiger, S. (2010) *The role of spirituality in the etiology and treatment of Complex Post Traumatic Stress Disorder.* California Southern University: ProQuest Dissertations Publishing. DPsychology thesis.

Ecker B. (2018) Flash Technique in EMDR: How and why it works. https://www.youtube.com/watch?v=m0ZiyerhzMc (accessed 13.9.18).

Elliott, R., Fischer, C.T. & Rennie, D.L. (1999) Evolving guidelines for publication of qualitative research studies in psychology and related fields. *British Journal of Clinical Psychology,* 38, 215-229.

Fontana, A. & Rosenheck, R. (2004) Trauma, change in strength of religious faith, and mental health service use among veterans treated for PTSD. https://www.ncbi.nlm.nih.gov/pubmed/15348973 Journal of Nervous and Mental Disorder, 192, 579-84.

Frankl, V. (2020) *The rediscovery of the human: Psychological writings of Viktor E. Frankel on the human in the image of the divine.* S. Cohen, Introduction. S. Cohen & L. Kosma, Translated. Melbourne, Australia: Hybrid.

Gall, T.L., Guirguis-Younger, M. . (2013) Religious and spiritual coping: Current theory and research. In Pargament, K.I., Exline, K., Jones, J., et al, editors. *APA Handbook of psychology, religion and spirituality.* Washington, D.C.: American Psychological Association, 349-364.

Goth, L. (undated, accessed 17.9.18) *EMDR and Christianity.*

https://maibergerinstitute.com/emdr-christianity

Harper, J. (2012) 84 percent of the world population has faith; a third are Christian - Washington Times Dec 23 2012. See also the full report: http://www.pewforum.org/.

Horst, F., Den Oudsten B., Zijlstra W., et al. (2017) Cognitive Behavioral Therapy vs. Eye Movement Desensitization and Reprocessing for treating panic disorder: A randomized controlled trial. Frontiers in Psychology: Clinical Health Psychologyg, 8, 1409-1418. doi: 10.3389/fpsyg.2017.01409.

Jeon, S.W., Han, C., Choi, J., Ko, Y., Yoon, H. & Kim, Y. (2017) Eye Movement Desensitization and Reprocessing to Facilitate Posttraumatic Growth: A Prospective Clinical Pilot Study on Ferry Disaster Survivors. *Clinical Psychopharmacology and Neuroscience, 15(4), 320-327.* doi: 10.9758/cpn.2017.15.4.320

Koenig, H., King, D., & Carson, V. editors. (2012). *Handbook of religion and health.* Oxford and New York, N.Y.: Oxford University Press.

Krystal, S., Prendergast, J. J., Krystal, P., Fenner, P., Shapiro, I., & Shapiro, K. (2002). Transpersonal psychology, Eastern nondual philosophy, and EMDR. In F. Shapiro (Ed.), *EMDR as an integrative psychotherapy approach: Experts of diverse orientations explore the paradigm prism* (pp. 319–339). American Psychological Association. https://doi.org/10.1037/10512-013

Logie, R. (2014) EMDR - more than just a therapy for PTSD? *The Psychologist,* 27, 512-516.

Loewenthal, K.M. (2007) *Religion, culture and mental health*. Cambridge: Cambridge University Press.

Loewenthal, K.M. (2013) Religion, Spirituality and Culture. In Pargament, K.I., Exline, K., Jones, J., et al, editors. *APA Handbook of psychology, religion and spirituality*. Washington, D.C.: American Psychological Association, 239-255.

Loewenthal, K.M. (2019) EMDR - Eye Movement Desensitization and Reprocessing Therapy and Religious Faith Among Orthodox Jewish (Haredi) Women. *Israel Journal of Psychiatry, 56(2),* 20-27.

Loewenthal, K.M. (2021) Religion, spirituality and recovery from trauma via EMDR therapy. Paper given at the conference of the *International Association for the Psychology of Religion* (online), August 2021.

Loewenthal, K.M., MacLeod, A.K., Goldblatt, V., Lubitsh, G. & Valentine, J.D. (2000) Comfort and joy: Religion, cognition and mood in individuals under stress. *Cognition and Emotion*, 14, 355-374.

Loewenthal, K.M., MacLeod, A.K., Goldblatt, V., et al. (2011) A gift that lasts? A prospective study of religion, cognition, mood and stress among Jews and Protestants. *World Cultural Psychiatry Research Review*, 6, 42-51.

Logie, R. (2014) EMDR - more than just a therapy for PTSD? *Psychologist*, 27, 512-516.

Manfield, P., Lovett, J., Engel, L., Manfield, D. (2017) Use of the Flash technique in EMDR therapy: Four case examples. *Journal of EMDR Practice and Research,* 11, 195-205.

Mayer, S. (2013). EMDR, spirituality, and healing in children. *Counselling and Spirituality / Counseling et spiritualité, 32*(1), 27–36.

National Institute for Health and Clinical Excellence (NICE) (2005). *Post traumatic stress disorder (PTSD).* London, 2005.

Nijdam, M.J, van der Meer, C.A.I., van Zuiden, M., Dashtgard, P., et al. (2018) Turning wounds into wisdom: Posttraumatic growth over the course of two types of trauma-focused psychotherapy in patients with PTSD. *Journal of Affective Disorders,* 227, 424-431. doi.org/10.1016/j.jad.2017.11.031

Panksepp, J. & Biven, L. (2012) A meditation on the affective neuroscientific view of human and animalian MindBrains. In Fotopoulou, A., Pfaff, D. & Conway, M.A. (Editors) *From the Couch to the Lab: Trends in Psychodynamic Neuroscience.* Oxford: Oxford University Press.

Pargament, K.I. (1997) *The psychology of religion and coping: Theory, research and practice.* New York, N.Y.: Guilford Press.

Pargament, K.I. (1998*)* Red flags and religious coping: identifying some religious warning signs among people in crisis. *Journal of Clinical Psychology,* 54, 77-89. https://www.ncbi.nlm.nih.gov/pubmed/9476711

Pargament, K.I. (2002) God help me: Advances in the psychology of religion and **coping**. *Archiv für Religionspsychologie / Archive for the Psychology of Religion,* 24, 48-63.

Pargament, K.I. & Exline, J.J. (2022) *Working with spiritual struggles in psychotherapy.* New York: Guilford.

Parnell, L. (1996) Eye movement desensitization and reprocessing (EMDR) and spiritual unfolding. *The Journal of Transpersonal Psychology*, 28 (2), 129-153.

Parnell, L. (2013) *Attachment-focused EMDR: Healing Relational trauma.* New York, NY: Norton.

Shapiro F. (2018). *Eye movement desensitization and reprocessing: Basic principles, protocols and procedures* (3rd edition). New York, N.Y.: Guilford Press.

Shaw, A., Joseph, S. & Linley, P.A. (2005) Religion, spirituality, and posttraumatic growth: a systematic review. *Mental Health, Religion & Culture, 8(1), 1-11.* https://doi.org/10.1080/1367467032000157981

Siegel, I.R. EMDR as a Transpersonal Therapy: A Trauma-Focused Approach to Awakening Consciousness. *Journal of EMDR Practice and Research*, 12(1), 24-43. DOI: 10.1891/1933-3196.12.1.24

Siegel, P., Warren, R., Wang, Z., et al. (2017). Less is more: Neural activity during very brief and clearly visible exposure to phobic stimuli. Human Brain Mapping, 38, 2466-2481. doi:10.1002/hbm.23533.

Soenke, M., Landau, M.J., & Greenberg, J. (2013) Sacred armour: Religion's roles as a buffer against the anxieties of life and the fear of death. In Pargament, K.I., Exline, K., Jones, J., et al, editors. *APA Handbook of psychology, religion and spirituality.* Washington, D.C.: American Psychological Association,105-122.

Stickgold, R. (2002) EMDR: A putative neurobiological mechanism of action. *Journal of Clinical Psychology,* 58, 61–75. https://doi.org/10.1002/jclp.1129

Tarakeshwar, N. (2013) What does it mean to be a Hindu? A review of common Hindu beliefs and practices and their implications for health. In Pargament, K.I., Exline, K., Jones, J., et al, editors. *APA Handbook of psychology, religion and spirituality.* Washington, D.C.: American Psychological Association,653-664.

Tedeschi, R.G. & Calhoun, L.G. (1996) The Posttraumatic Growth Inventory: measuring the positive legacy of trauma. *Journal of Traumatic Stress*, 9(3), 455-471. doi:10.1007/BF02103658

Turpin, R.C. (1999) *An exploration of reported transpersonal/spiritual experiences during and after movement desensitization and reprocessing (EMDR) treatment of traumatic memories.* California Institute of Integral Studies: DPsychology Dissertation.

Valiente-Gomez, A., Moreno-Alcázar, A., Devi Treen, D. et al. (2017). EMDR beyond PTSD: A Systematic Literature Review. *Frontiers in Psychology*, 26 September 2017. https://doi.org/10.3389/fpsyg.2017.01668

World Health Organization. (2013) *Guidelines for the management of conditions specifically related to stress.* Geneva.

APPENDIX

Kate Miriam Loewenthal: complete list of published academic articles.
This list is shown to give an indication of my research interests and how they changed.

1. K.Loewenthal: How are first impressions formed? *Psychological Reports*, 1967, 21, 834-836.

2. K.Loewenthal: The development of codes in public and private language. *Psychonomic Science*, 1967, 8, 449-450.

3. K.Loewenthal: The effects of understanding from the audience on language behaviour. *British Journal of Social and Clinical Psychology*, 1968, 7, 247-252.

4. K.Loewenthal & J.Briem: Immediate recall of nominalisations and adjectivalisations.*Psychonomic Science*, 1968, 11, 209-210.

5. K.Loewenthal: Semantic features and communicability of words of different form-class. *Psychonomic Science*, 1969, 17, 79-80.

6. K.Loewenthal: A study of imperfectly acquired vocabulary. *British Journal of Psychology*, 1971, 62, 225-233.

7. K.Loewenthal: Effects of understanding from the audience on language behaviour. In S.Moscovici (ed) *Readings in Sociopsycholinguistics*, Mouton,1972.

8. K.Loewenthal & B.Kostrevski: The effects of training in written communication on verbal skills. *British Journal of Educational Psychology*, 1973, 43, 82-86.

9. K.Loewenthal & G.Gibbs: Word familiarity and retention. *Quarterly Journal of Experimental Psychology*, 1974, 26, 15-25.

10. K.M.Loewenthal: Property. *European Journal of Social Psychology*, 1974, 6, 73-81.

11. K.Loewenthal: Psychology and Religion: comments on Giles, Jones, Horton and Lay. *Bulletin of the British Psychological Society*, 1975, 28, 349-350.

12. K.Loewenthal: Handwriting and self-presentation. *Journal of Social Psychology*, 1975, 96, 267-270.

13. K.Loewenthal & P.Bick: Silence and role uncertainty. *Journal of Social Psychology*, 1976, 99, 151.

14. K.Loewenthal: What is the unconscious? *Learn*, 1979, 3, 36.

15. K.Loewenthal: Exams: how to cope with stress. *Learn*, 1979, 7, 7-9.

16. K.Loewenthal: The UFO phenomenon. *New Society*, 1979, 47, 241-2.

17. K.Loewenthal: What does handwriting tell us about personality? *New Society*, 1980, 51, 544-5.

18. S.Tahta, M.Wood & K.Loewenthal: Foreign accents: factors relating to transfer of accent from the first language to a second language. *Language and Speech*, 1981, 24, 265-72.

19. S.Tahta, M.Wood & K.Loewenthal: Age changes in the ability to replicate foreign pronunciation and intonation. *Language and Speech*, 1981, 24, 367-72.

20. K.Loewenthal: Family planning: Jewish attitudes. In T.Gurary (ed) *Aura: a reader on Jewish Womanhood.* New York: Lubavitch, 1985.

21. K.Loewenthal: Handwriting as a guide to character. In M.Harris & D.MacKenzie-Davey (eds) *Judging People*, McGraw-Hill, 1982.

22. K.M.Loewenthal: Jewish attitudes to family planning. *Jewish Chronicle*, August 1982.

23. K.Loewenthal & D.Bull: Imitation of foreign sounds: what is the effect of age? *Language and Speech*, 1984, 27, 95-98.

24. K.Loewenthal: Attribution of religious commitment: different accounts by the religious and the nonreligious. *Journal of Social Psychology*, 1985, 125, 519-520.

25. K.Loewenthal: Unstructured groups in undergraduate social psychology teaching. *Psychology Teaching*, 1985.

26. K.Loewenthal: Factors affecting religious commitment. *Journal of Social Psychology*, 1986, 125-126.

27. K.Loewenthal: Religious development and experience in Habad-hasidic women. *Journal of Psychology and Judaism*, 1988, 12, 5-20.

28. K.Loewenthal: The shape of Jews to come. In C.Shindler (ed) *Fourth Jacob Sonntag Memorial Symposium, Jewish Quarterly*, 1989, 133, 34-43.

29. K.M.Loewenthal: The happiness of the Anglo-Jewish woman. *HaMaor*, 1989, 18-21.

30. K.Loewenthal: Marriage and religious commitment: the case of hasidic women. *Religion Today*, 1988, 5, 8-10.

31. K.Eames & K.Loewenthal: Non-content factors in the assessment of essays; handwriting and the judge's expertise. *Journal of Social Psychology*, 1990, 130, 831-834.

32. K.Loewenthal: Judaism and Feminism. In P.Ginsbury (ed) *L'Eylah: special issue on Feminism*, London,1991.

33. M.James & K.Loewenthal: Handwriting stereotypes for the judgment of depression. *Journal of Social Psychology*, 1991, 131, 747-748

34. A.Jarrett & K.M.Loewenthal: Employer's social judgments based on handwriting and

typeface. *Journal of Social Psychology*,1991, 131, 749-750

35. K.Loewenthal: Depression, Melancholy and Judaism. *International Journal for the Psychology of Religion, 1992, 2, 101-108.*

36. K.Loewenthal, K.Eames, C.Loewenthal, V.Goldblatt, V.Amos and S.Mullarkey) Levels of wellbeing and distress in orthodox Jewish men and women. *Journal of Psychology and Judaism,* 1993, 16, 225-233.

37. K.Loewenthal: Religion, stress and distress. *Religion Today*, 1993, 8, 14-16.

38. K.Loewenthal & N.Cornwall: Religiosity and perceived control of life events *International Journal for the Psychology of Religion,*1993, 3, 39-46.

39. K.M.Loewenthal & V.Goldblatt: Family size and depressive symptoms in orthodox Jewish women. *Journal of Psychiatric Research*, 1993, 27,3-10.

40. K.M.Loewenthal: Judaism and Psychoanalysis, *L'Eylah,* 1993, 35, 42-43.

41. K.Loewenthal, V. Goldblatt, V. Amos & S.Mullarkey: Some correlates of wellbeing and distress in Anglo-Jewish women. In L.Brown (ed)*Religion, Personality and Mental Health.*New York: Springer-Verlag, 1993.

42. K.M.Loewenthal, V.Goldblatt & others: Gender and depression in Anglo-Jewry. *Psychological Medicine*, 1995, 25, 1051-1063.

43. K.M.Loewenthal & C.Bradley: Immunisation uptake and doctors' perceptions of uptake in a minority group: implications for interventions. *Psychology, Health and Medicine*, 1996, 1, 223-230.

44. S.Hamid & K.M.Loewenthal: Inferring gender from handwriting in Urdu and English. *Journal of Social Psychology*, 1996, 136, 778-782.

45. K.M.Loewenthal: Religious beliefs about illness. *International Journal for the Psychology of Religion*, 1997, 7, 173-176.

46. B.Grady & K.M.Loewenthal: Features associated with speaking in tongues (Glossolalia). *British Journal of Medical Psychology*, 1997, 70, 185-191.

47. K.M.Loewenthal: Stress and distress in orthodox-Jewish men and women. *British Psychological Society, Bulletin of the Psychology of Women Section*, 1996, 18, 6-11.

48. K.M. Loewenthal, V.Goldblatt & others: The social circumstances of anxiety among Anglo-Jews. *Journal of Affective Disorders*, 1997, 46, 87-94.

49. K.M. Loewenthal, V.Goldblatt & others: (1997) The costs and benefits of boundary maintenance: Stress, religion and culture among Jews in Britain. *Social Psychiatry and Psychiatric Epidemiology*, 32, 200-207.

50. A.Kose & K.M.Loewenthal: Conversion motifs in British converts to Islam. *International Journal for Psychology of Religion*, 10, 101-110, 2000

51. K.M.Loewenthal: Religion and Depression in the Jewish context.

52. K.M.Loewenthal: Review article on The Unconscious at Work: Individual and Organizational Stress in the Human Services, edited by A. Obholzer & V.Roberts. *Human Relations*, 49 , 1998.

53. K.M.Loewenthal: Invited review of *Psychiatry and Religion*, edited by D. Bhugra. *Psychological Medicine,* 27, 1450-1452, 1998.

54. K.M.Loewenthal: Haredi women, Haredi men, stress and distress. *Israel Journal of Psychiatry,* 35, 217-224, 1998.

55. K.M.Loewenthal: Religious issues in mental health among minority groups: Issues in Great Britain in the 1990s. *International Journal for the Psychology of Religion.*

56. S.Dein & K.M.Loewenthal: Editorial: Mental health and religion. *Mental Health, Religion and Culture*, 1, 5-10, 1998.

57. S.Dein & K.M.Loewenthal: Holy healing: The growth of religious and spiritual therapies. *Mental Health, Religion and Culture*, 1, 85-90, 1998

58. M.Cinnirella & K.M.Loewenthal: Religious and ethnic group influences on beliefs about mental illness: A qualitative interview study. *British Journal of Medical Psychology,* 72, 505-524, 1999.

59. K.M.Loewenthal: Religious issues and their psychological aspects. In K.Bhui & D.Olajide (eds) *Cross Cultural Mental Health Services: Contemporary Issues in Service Provision*. London: W.B. Saunders, 1999.

60. S.Dein & K.M.Loewenthal: The millennium and mental health. *Mental Health, Religion and Culture*, 2, 5-8, 1999.

61. K.M.Loewenthal & M.Cinnirella: Beliefs about the efficacy of religious, medical and psychotherapeutic interventions for depression and

schizophrenia among different cultural-religious groups in Great Britain. *Transcultural Psychiatry*, 36, 491-504, 1999.

62. S.Dein & K.M.Loewenthal: Mysticism and psychiatry. *Mental Health, Religion and Culture*, 2, 101-104, 1999.

63. K.M.Loewenthal, M.W.Eysenck, D.Harris, G.Lubitsh, T.Gorton & G. Keinan: Job dysfunction and distress in airline pilots in relation to contextually-assessed stress. *Stress Medicine*, 16, 179-183, 2000.

64. M.Yossifova & K.M.Loewenthal: Religion and the judgement of obsessionality. *Mental Health, Religion and Culture*, 2, 145-152, 1999.

65. K.M.Loewenthal, A.K.MacLeod, V. Goldblatt, G.Lubitsh & J.D.Valentine: Comfort and Joy: Religion, cognition and mood in individuals under stress. *Cognition and Emotion*, 14, 355-374, 2000.

66. K.M.Loewenthal, A.K.MacLeod & M.Cinnirella:Are women more religious than men? Gender differences in religious activity among different religious groups in the UK. *Personality and Individual Differences*, 32, 133-139, 2001.

67. K.M.Loewenthal with M.Brooke-Rogers: Culturally and religiously sensitive psychological help - from a Jewish perspective. In S.King-Spooner & C.Newnes (eds) *Spirituality and Psychotherapy*. Ross-on-Wye: PCCS Books, 2001

68. K.M.Loewenthal, M.Cinnirella, G. Evdoka & P.Murphy: Faith conquers all? Beliefs about the role of religious factors in coping with depression among different cultural-religious groups in the UK. *British Journal of Medical Psychology*, 74, 293-303, 2001.

69. Z.Kamal & K.M.Loewenthal: Suicide beliefs and behaviour among young Muslims and Hindus in the UK. *Mental Health, Religion and Culture*, 5, 111-118, 2002.

70. K.M.Loewenthal, A.K.MacLeod, S.Cook, M.J.Lee & V.Goldblatt (2002) Tolerance for depression : Are there cultural and gender differences? *Journal of Psychiatric and Mental Health Nursing*, 9, 681-688.

71. K.M.Loewenthal: A contemporary interface between religion and psychotherapy. *Journal of Judaism and Civilisation*, 4, 64-79, 2002.

72. K.M.Loewenthal & M.Cinnirella: (2003) Religious issues in ethnic minority mental health with special reference to schizophrenia in Afro-Caribbeans in Britain: a systematic review. In D.Ndegwa & D.Olajide (editors) *Main Issues in Mental Health and Race.* London: Ashgate

73. K.M.Loewenthal, A.K.MacLeod, S.Cook, M.J.Lee & V.Goldblatt: Beliefs about alcohol among UK Jews and Protestants: Do they fit the alcohol-depression hypothesis? *Social Psychiatry and Psychiatric Epidemiology,* 38, 122-127, 2003.

74. Lindsey, C., Frosh, S., Loewenthal, K.M. and Spitzer, E. Emotional and behaviour disorders among strictly-orthodox Jewish pre-school children, *Clinical Child Psychology and Psychiatry,* 8, 459-472, 2003.

75. K.M.Loewenthal, A.K.MacLeod, S.Cook, M.J.Lee & V.Goldblatt: (2003)The suicide beliefs of Jews and Protestants in the UK: How do they differ? *Israel Journal of Psychiatry*, 40, 174-181.

76. K.Loewenthal: A case of new identity: Detecting the forces facing Jewish identity and community. In J.Boyd (Editor) *Jewish Identity and Community*, Jerusalem: Hebrew University, 2003.

77. K.M.Loewenthal, A.K.MacLeod, S.Cook, M.J.Lee & V.Goldblatt (2003) Drowning your sorrows? Attitudes towards alcohol in UK Jews and Protestants: A thematic analysis. *International Journal of Social Psychiatry,* 49, 204-215.

78. M.Brooke Rogers & K.M.Loewenthal. Religion, Identity and Mental Health (2003) Perceived interactions within a multi-dimensional framework. *Social Psychology Review,* 5, 43-81.

79. L Glinert, K.M.Loewenthal & V Goldblatt (2003) Guarding the Tongue: A thematic analysis of gossip control strategies among orthodox Jewish women, *Journal of Multilingual & Multicultural Development,* 24, 513-524.

80. K.M.Loewenthal & M.Brooke Rogers (2004). Culture sensitive support groups: how are they perceived and how do they work? *International Journal of Social Psychiatry,* 50, 227-240.

81. Frosh, S., Loewenthal, K.M., Lindsey, C. & Spitzer, E. (2005) Prevalence of emotional and behavioural disorders among strictly orthodox Jewish children in London, *Clinical Child Psychology and Psychiatry,* 10, 351-368.

82. Loewenthal, K.M. Mental Health and Religion. In D.M.Wulff (editor) *Psychology and Religion.* Oxford: Oxford University Press.

83. Loewenthal, K.M. (2005) Strictly Orthodox Jews and their relations with psychiatry and psychotherapy. *Transcultural Psychiatry Section World Psychiatric Association Newsletter,* 23(1), 20-24.

84. Rogers, M.B., Lewis, C.A., Loewenthal, K.M., Cinnirella, M., & Ansari, H (2005) Aspects of Terrorism and Martyrdom: Seminar One – What roles are played religious beliefs and identity in supporting views of

violent activists as terrorists or martyrs? In Lewis, C.A., Rogers, M.B, Loewenthal, K.M., Cinnirella, M., Amlot, R. & Ansari, H. (Editors) *Proceedings of the British Psychological Society Seminar Series Aspects of Terrorism and Martyrdom. eCOMMUNITY: International Journal of Mental Health and Addiction.*

85. Gummer, C. & Loewenthal, K.M. (2005) British Christian views of suicide bombers. In Lewis, C.A., Rogers, M.B, Loewenthal, K.M., Cinnirella, M., Amlot, R. & Ansari, H. (Editors) *Proceedings of the British Psychological Society Seminar Series Aspects of Terrorism and Martyrdom. eCOMMUNITY: International Journal of Mental Health and Addiction.*

86. Amlot, R., Loewenthal, K.M., Lewis, C.A., Rogers, M.B., Cinnirella, M., & Ansari, H (2005) Aspects of Terrorism and Martyrdom: Seminar Two – What factors influence the process of embracing concepts of terrorism and martyrdom? ? In Lewis, C.A., Rogers, M.B, Loewenthal, K.M., Cinnirella, M., Amlot, R. & Ansari, H. (Editors) *Proceedings of the British Psychological Society Seminar Series Aspects of Terrorism and Martyrdom. eCOMMUNITY: International Journal of Mental Health and Addiction.*

87. Ansari, H., Cinnirella, M., Rogers, M.B., Loewenthal, K.M. & (2005) Perceptions of martyrdom and terrorism among British Muslims. ? In Lewis, C.A., Rogers, M.B, Loewenthal, K.M., Cinnirella, M., Amlot, R. & Ansari, H. (Editors) *Proceedings of the British Psychological Society Seminar Series Aspects of Terrorism and Martyrdom. eCOMMUNITY: International Journal of Mental Health and Addiction.*

88. Lewis, C.A., Rogers, M.B., Amlot, R., Loewenthal, K.M., Cinnirella, M., & Ansari, H (2005) Aspects of Terrorism and Martyrdom: Seminar Three – Exploring organisational contributory factors and socio-religious outcomes of terrorism and martyrdom? ? In Lewis, C.A., Rogers, M.B

Loewenthal, K.M., Cinnirella, M., Amlot, R. & Ansari, H. (Editors) *Proceedings of the British Psychological Society Seminar Series Aspects of Terrorism and Martyrdom. eCOMMUNITY: International Journal of Mental Health and Addiction.*

89. Loewenthal, K.M. (2006) Orthodox Judaism: Issues and features for psychotherapy. In T.Dowd & S.Nielsen (editors) *Exploration of the Psychologies in Religion.* New York: Springer.

90. Loewenthal, K.M. (2007) Spirituality and Cultural Psychiatry. In D.Bhugra & K.Bhui (editors) *Textbook of Cultural Psychiatry.* Cambridge: Cambridge University Press.

91. Loewenthal, K.M. (2006) Strictly orthodox Jews and their relations with psychotherapy and psychiatry. *World Cultural Psychiatry Research Review, 1, Special Issue on Culture, Spirituality and Mental Health.*

92. Leavey,G., Loewenthal, K.M. & King, M. (2007) Challenges to sanctuary: the clergy as a resource for mental health care in the community. *Social Science and Medicine,* 65, 548-559.

93. Rogers, M.B., Loewenthal, K.M., Lewis, C.A., Amlot, R., Cinnirella, M., Ansari, H. (2007) The Role of Religious Fundamentalism in Terrorist Violence: A Social Psychological Analysis. *International Review of Psychiatry,* 19, 253-262. (IF 1.733)

94. Inaba, K. & Loewenthal, K.M. (2008) Religion and Altruism. In Clarke, P. (editor) *Oxford Handbook of the Sociology of Religion.* Oxford: Oxford University Press.

95. Loewenthal, K.M. & Rogers, M.B. (2008) Culturally and religiously sensitive help: from a Jewish perspective. *Journal of Clinical Psychology, Counselling and Psychotherapy,* 8, 39-53.

96. Loewenthal, K. (2009) Psychology of Religion. In Clarke, P. & Beyer, P. (eds) *The World's Religions*, pp 867-889. London: Routledge.

97. Loewenthal, K.M. (2009) The Alcohol-Depression Hypothesis: Gender and the Prevalence of Depression among Jews. In L. Sher (ed) *Comorbidity of Depression and Alcohol Use Disorders.* Nova Science Publishers. (pp 31-40)

98. Loewenthal, K.M. (2009) Spirituality and religion: friends or foes? Views from the orthodox Jewish community. *Royal College of Psychiatrists Spirituality and Psychiatry Special Interest Group Newsletter, Winter 2009.*

99. Bradley C, Loewenthal K, Woodcock A and McMillan C (2009) Development of the diabetes treatment satisfaction questionnaire (DTSQ) for teenagers and parents: the DTSQ-Teen and the DTSQ-Parent. Diabetologia 52: (Suppl 1) S397, Abstract 1013.

100. Loewenthal,K.M., MacLeod, A.K., Goldblatt, V., Lubitsh, G. & Valentine, J.D. (2011) A gift that lasts? A prospective study of religion, cognition, mood and stress among Jews and Protestants. *World Cultural Psychiatry Research Review*, 6, 42-51.

101. Gummer, C. & Loewenthal, K.M. (2012) British Christian views of suicide bombers. In Lewis, C.A., Rogers, M.B, Loewenthal, K.M., Cinnirella, M., Amlot, R. & Ansari, H. (Editors) *Aspects of Terrorism and Martyrdom: Dying for Good, Dying for God*. Lampeter : The Edwin Mellen Press

102. Social identity and beliefs about martyrdom and terrorism amongst British Muslims. Cinnirella, M., Lewis, C., Ansari, H., Loewenthal, K., Brooke-Rogers, M. & Amlot, R. (2012) *Aspects of Terrorism and Martyrdom: Dying for Good, Dying for God (Volumes 1, 2, 3)*. Lewis, C. A.,

Rogers, M. B., Amlot, R., Loewenthal, K. M., Cinnirella, M. & Ansari, H. (eds.). Lampeter: The Edwin Mellen Press.

103. Loewenthal, K.M. (2010) The case for narrative. Special Issue on J.A. Belzen (2010) *"Towards a Cultural Psychology of Religion"*, New York: Springer. *Mental Health, Religion and Culture*, 13, 391-395.

104. Loewenthal, K.M. & Lewis, C.A. (2011) Mental health, religion and culture. *The Psychologist*, 24, 256-259.

105. Dein, S., Lewis, C.A. & Loewenthal, K.M. (2011) Psychiatrists' views on the place of religion in psychiatry: An introduction to this special issue of *Mental Health, Religion and Culture*. *Mental Health, Religion and Culture*, 14, 1-9.

106. Loewenthal, K.M. (2011) Changing ways of doing things: an autobiographical account of some of my experiences in the psychology of religion. In J.Belzen (Editor) *Psychology of Religion in Autobiography*, pp133-154. New York: Springer.

107. Band, M., Dein, S. & Loewenthal, K.M. (2011) Religiosity, Coping and Suicidality within the Religious Zionist Community of Israel. A Thematic Qualitative Analysis. *Mental Health, Religion and Culture*, 14, 1031-1048.

108. Al-Solaim, L. & Loewenthal, K.M. (2011) Religion and obsessive-compulsive disorder (OCD) among young Muslim women in Saudi Arabia. *Mental Health, Religion and Culture*, 14, 169-182.

109. Loewenthal, K.M. (2012) Mental health and mental health care for Jews in the diaspora, with particular reference to the UK. *Israel Journal of Psychiatry*, 49, 159-166.

110. Loewenthal, Kate (2012) Spirit possession – Jews don't do that, so they? Royal College of Psychiatrists, *Spirituality and Psychiatry Special Interest Group Newsletter,* 34, 1-7.

111. Loewenthal. Kate M. (2012) Charity. In David Leeming (editor) *Encylopedia of Psychology and Religion.* Springer.*

112. Loewenthal. Kate M. (2012) Conscience. In David Leeming (editor) *Encylopedia of Psychology and Religion.* Springer.*

113. Loewenthal. Kate M. (2012) Depression. In David Leeming (editor) *Encylopedia of Psychology and Religion.* Springer.*

114. Loewenthal. Kate M. (2012) Hasidism. In David Leeming (editor) *Encylopedia of Psychology and Religion.* Springer.*

115. Loewenthal. Kate M. (2012) Psychology. In David Leeming (editor) *Encylopedia of Psychology and Religion.* Springer.*

116. Loewenthal. Kate M. (2012) Psychosis. In David Leeming (editor) *Encylopedia of Psychology and Religion.* Springer.*

117. Loewenthal. Kate M. (2012) Psychotherapy and Religion. In David Leeming (editor) *Encylopedia of Psychology and Religion.* Springer.*

118. Loewenthal. Kate M. (2012) Zionism. In David Leeming (editor) *Encylopedia of Psychology and Religion.* Springer.*

119. Bayes, JEB. & Loewenthal, KM (2013) How do Jewish teachings relate to beliefs about depression in the strictly orthodox Jewish community? *Mental Health, Religion and Culture,* 16, 852-862.

120. Dein, S. & Loewenthal, K.M. (2013) The mental health benefits and costs of Sabbath observance among orthodox Jews. *Journal of Religion and Health*, 52, 1382-1390.

121. Loewenthal, K.M. (2013) Religion, Spirituality and Culture. In K.I.Pargament, J.Exline, J.Jones, A.Mahoney, E.Shafranske (Editors), APA Handbook of Psychology, Religion and Spirituality. Washington, DC: American Psychological Association.

122. Loewenthal, K.M. (2014) Religion, identity and mental health. In R.Jaspal & G.Breakwell (Editors) *Identity Process Theory: Identity, Social Action and Social Change.* Cambridge: Cambridge University Press.

123. Loewenthal, K.M. (2014) Addiction: Alcohol and substance abuse in Judaism. *Religions: Special Issue: Religion and Addiction, 5, 972-984* (doi: 10.3390/rel5040972) (http://www.mdpi.com/2077-1444/5/4/972/pdf)

124. Loewenthal, K.M. (2015). Psychiatry and Religion. In: James D. Wright (editor-in-chief), *International Encyclopedia of the Social & Behavioral Sciences, 2nd edition, Vol 19.* Oxford: Elsevier. pp. 307–312.

*Chapters numbered 111-118 above revised and updated 2015.

125. Loewenthal, K.M. (2015): Psychological perspectives on religion and religiosity. *Mental Health, Religion & Culture*, DOI: http://dx.doi.org/10.1080/13674676.2015.1057114

126. Loewenthal, K.M. (2015) Religious ritual and well-being. In Ben-Avie, M., Ives, Y. & Loewenthal, K.M.. (editors) *Jewish Social Values and Contemporary Social Problems.* New York: Springer.

127. Leavey, G., Loewenthal, K.M. & King, M. (2016) Locating the social origins of mental illness: The explanatory models of mental illness from

different ethnic and faith backgrounds. *Journal of Religion and Health,* published online (DOI 10 1007/s10943-016-0191-1)

128. Loewenthal, K.M. & Solaim, L.S. (2016) Religious Identity, Challenge, and Clothing: Women's head and hair covering in Islam and Judaism. *Journal of Empirical Theology,* 29, 160-170.

129. Loewenthal. Kate M. (2018) Charity. In David Leeming (editor) *Encylopedia of Psychology and Religion.* Springer.

130. Loewenthal. Kate M. (2018) Conscience. In David Leeming (editor) *Encylopedia of Psychology and Religion.* Springer.

131. Loewenthal. Kate M. (2018) Depression. In David Leeming (editor) *Encylopedia of Psychology and Religion.* Springer.

132. Loewenthal. Kate M. (2018) Psychology. In David Leeming (editor) *Encylopedia of Psychology and Religion.* Springer.

133. Loewenthal. Kate M. (2018) Psychosis. In David Leeming (editor) *Encylopedia of Psychology and Religion.* Springer.

134. Loewenthal. Kate M. (2018) Psychotherapy and Religion. In David Leeming (editor) *Encylopedia of Psychology and Religion.* Springer.*

135. Loewenthal. Kate M. (2018) Zionism. In David Leeming (editor) *Encylopedia of Psychology and Religion.* Springer.

136. Perry, A., Gardener, C., Dove, J., Eiger, Y., Loewenthal, K.M. (2018) Improving mental health knowledge of the Charedi Orthodox Jewish community in North London: A partnership project. *International Journal of Social Psychiatry,* 64, 235-247.

137. Loewenthal. Kate M. (2019) Modest dress: the rules, the controversies and the experiences. In P.Wexler (Editor) *Jewish Spirituality and Social Transformation,* pp99-112. New York: Crossroad Publishing.

138. Loewenthal. Kate M. (2019) The OCD - religion package: might it relate to the rise of spirituality? *Mental Health, Religion & Culture*, online https://doi.org/10.1080/13674676.2018.1447554

139. Lewis, C.A. & Loewenthal, K.M. (2018) Editorial: Religion and obsessionality: Obsessive actions and religious practices. *Mental Health, Religion & Culture,* 21 (2), 117–122. https://doi.org/10.1080/13674676.2018.1481192

140. Loewenthal, K.M. (2019) EMDR - Eye Movement Desensitization and Reprocessing therapy and religious faith among orthodox Jewish (*hareidi*) women**.** *Israel Journal of Psychiatry & Related Sciences, 56 (2), 20-27.* \מס בקרב נשים יהודיות חרדיות טיפול בתנועות עיניים ואתונה דתית\.

141. Loewenthal, K.M. (2019) Intersections among Religion, Culture, Gender, and Mental Health. In J.Mena & K.Quina (Editors) *Integrating Multiculturalism and Intersectionality Into the Psychology Curriculum.* Washington, DC: American Psychological Association, pp 143-156.

142. Dein, S., Loewenthal, K., Lewis, C.A. & Pargament, K.I. (2020) COVID-19, mental health and religion: an agenda for future research. *Mental Health, Religion & Culture,* 23 (1), 1–9.

143. Loewenthal, K.M. & Marcus, B. (2020) Jewish Stereotypes in Psychiatric Diagnosis and Treatment. In Moffic, H.S., Peteet, J.R., Hankir, A., Seeman**,** M.V. (Eds.) *Anti-Semitism and Psychiatry: Recognition, Prevention, and Interventions.* Springer.

144. Loewenthal, K.M.(2021) Anti-semitism in psychology. In Newnes, C. & Golding, L. (Eds). *Racism in Psychology* London and New York Routledge.

145. Loewenthal, K., Lewis, C.A., Dein, S. & Pargament, K.I. (2022) Editorial: Religious/spiritual coping and adversity. *Mental Health, Religion & Culture*, (In press)

146. Loewenthal, K. (2022) Religious change and posttraumatic growth following trauma therapy: A systematic review. *Mental Health, Religion & Culture*, (In press)

www.ingramcontent.com/pod-product-compliance
Lightning Source LLC
Chambersburg PA
CBHW071351300426
44114CB00030B/1993